FROM THE EDITORS OF
Arthritis Today

The Essential Guide to **Arthritis**
Medications

Prescription and Over-the-Counter
Treatments for Your Joint Pain
[FROM **A** TO **Z**]

CHIEF MEDICAL EDITOR: JOHN H. KLIPPEL, MD
PRESIDENT AND CEO, THE ARTHRITIS FOUNDATION

The Essential Guide to **Arthritis** **Medications**

Prescription and Over-the-Counter
Treatments for Your Joint Pain
[FROM **A** TO **Z**]

FROM THE EDITORS OF
Arthritis Today

CHIEF MEDICAL EDITOR: JOHN H. KLIPPEL, MD
PRESIDENT AND CEO, THE ARTHRITIS FOUNDATION

PUBLISHED BY

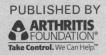

ARTHRITIS FOUNDATION®
Take Control. We Can Help.™

The Essential Guide to Arthritis Medications

From the experts you trust at *Arthritis Today*

An Official Publication of the Arthritis Foundation

Copyright 2006
Arthritis Foundation
1330 West Peachtree Street
Suite 100
Atlanta, GA 30309

Library of Congress Card Catalog Number: 2005932483

ISBN: 0-912423-48-X

Printed in the United States

This book was conceived, designed and produced by the
Arthritis Foundation. The mission of the Arthritis Foundation
is to improve lives through leadership in the prevention, control
and cure of arthritis and related diseases.

Editorial Director: BETHANY AFSHAR

Art Director and Cover Designer: TRACIE BULLIS

Contents

Chapter *I*

A Primer on Arthritis and Its Treatment

Chapter *II*

Taking Medications: What You Need to Know

Chapter III

Drugs to Treat Arthritis and Related Conditions

When you can't get your medication

On September 30, 2004, the unexpected happened: One of the most popular pain relievers of all time – rofecoxib (*Vioxx*) – was withdrawn from the market. Many people who used *Vioxx* to ease arthritis pain were left in shock. Some were left with bottles of unused pills. All were left wondering, what's next?

Around the same time, many people who relied on weekly injections of the disease-modifying drug methotrexate began having difficulty finding their drug. The problem, it turned out, was that the plant that manufactured the majority of the U.S. supply of methotrexate had temporarily closed for an upgrade. With that source of methotrexate shut down, the supply quickly dwindled. Many people searched for pharmacies that still had a supply of the injectable liquid; others began to examine their other treatment options.

While the two incidents are much different, the result was much the same: people were unable (in the case of methotrexate, temporarily; in the case of *Vioxx,* permanently) to get the drugs they had trusted.

Unfortunately, the situation is not that uncommon. Just two years before the methotrexate shortage started, for example, a shortage of the biologic agent etanercept (*Enbrel*) prompted the Seattle-based biotechnology company Immunex to send letters to the 84,000 *Enbrel* users, warning them of delays – ranging from a few days to a few weeks – in receiving their prescription. Some 20,000 other would-be *Enbrel* users were placed on a waiting list to receive the drug.

Numerous drugs, including the nonsteroidal anti-inflammatory drug bromfenac (*Duract*) and COX-2 inhibitor valdecoxib (*Bextra*) have been pulled from the market in recent years.

What gives?

There are many reasons a drug may be in short supply and/or pulled off the market completely.

Drug shortages are usually temporary and may have a number of causes. In *Enbrel*'s case, the manufacturer could not keep up with the greater-than-expected demand for the then relatively new agent. Producing more *Enbrel* meant first building a new manufacturing plant and the approval of that plant by the Federal Drug Administration (FDA) – a process that ultimately took a couple of years. Other reasons for shortages include FDA-mandated repairs or upgrades of manufacturing facilities (as was the case with methotrexate), mergers of companies manufacturing the drug and difficulty obtaining raw materials to produce the drug.

For drug withdrawals, the reason is often safety-related. Even after drugs are approved by the FDA, scientists continue to discover and collect information about them. Often, what they find is good – for example, a drug used for rheumatoid arthritis may also be helpful for other forms of the disease – but sometimes unexpected dangers are uncovered. In the case of *Vioxx*, for example, a large study suggested that adults taking the drug for more than 18 months had a 50 percent greater risk of heart attacks and sudden cardiac death than those taking a similar drug, celecoxib (*Celebrex*). That finding ultimately prompted *Vioxx*'s maker Merck to withdraw it from the market.

Regardless of the reasons your drug is gone or in short supply, the result is usually frustration, uncertainty and the need for changes in treatment. What do you do when you can't get your medication? Here are a few suggestions.

Check around – When methotrexate was in short supply, many patients were able to continue the drug by checking with mail-order pharmacies and scouring drug stores in their area.

Check with your doctor – When a shortage is the issue, your doctor may have some reserve supplies of the medication you need. When a drug is not available – because of a temporary shortage or permanent withdrawal – your doctor will work with you to find the best alternative. In some cases, a similar drug is available. For example, many *Vioxx* users switched to *Celebrex*, another drug in the class called cyclooxygenase-2 (COX-2) inhibitors. Many of those who were unable to get injectable methotrexate switched to oral methotrexate – which may not have been as effective as the injection, but was sufficient short term – until they were able to get their injections again.

Do your research – Is the shortage temporary or permanent? You can find out by visiting the Web sites of the FDA (www.fda.gov) or the American Society of Health-System Pharmacists (www.ashp.org). Both sites provide a listing of drugs in short supply along with the reason for the shortage. The ASHP site also offers suggestions for drugs that might be taken in place of the one in short supply.

As this edition of *The Essential Guide to Arthritis Medications* went to press, all of the drugs included were either available or expected to be available in sufficient quantities. But, as we learned from *Vioxx*, that can change quickly.

Fortunately, with all of the many drugs on the market – and new ones being developed – chances are you can find one that works for you, even if the one you've relied on is suddenly unavailable.

What to Do with Leftovers

Your medication is pulled from the market just three days after you purchased a 90-day supply. Can you continue to take the drug, or are you simply out of your hard-earned cash? The answer, in most cases, is neither. While you should never take a drug that has been pulled from the market, that doesn't mean you have to eat the cost. Speak to your doctor or pharmacist about what you can do with the drug. *Vioxx*'s manufacturer, for example, reimbursed prescription holders for their unused medications.

Acknowledgments

The Essential Guide to Arthritis Medications is written for people who have arthritis or other related diseases, as well as for their friends, family and loved ones. Bringing this book to completion was a team effort, including the significant contributions of dedicated physicians, healthcare professionals, Arthritis Foundation volunteers, writers, editors, designers and Arthritis Foundation staff.

Special acknowledgments should go to Mary Anne Dunkin, who compiled and wrote the text based on the annual *Drug Guide* published in *Arthritis Today* magazine. Dunkin is the author of the books *The Arthritis Foundation's Guide to Managing Your Arthritis* and *All You Need to Know About Back Pain*. Dunkin is former Senior Editor of *Arthritis Today* magazine. In addition, we would like to acknowledge Donna Rae Siegfried, Medical Editor of *Arthritis Today*, and Robin Yamakawa, Manager of Custom Publishing, Arthritis Foundation, for their assistance on this book.

The chief medical editor of the book was John H. Klippel, MD, the President and CEO of the Arthritis Foundation.

This book's content was developed with the help of an independent panel of medical experts, including medical doctors, other health professionals and researchers, who study, research and administer these drugs every day. These people are considered some of the foremost experts on arthritis and related drugs in this country, perhaps in the world. They volunteered their time to guide us through the creation of this book's content, as well to review the final content. They worked from the Food and Drug Administration-approved package inserts for each drug and pored over those complex documents, distilling the most pertinent information to bring to you in a format you can easily use and understand.

We would like to acknowledge these experts and thank them for the hard work and time they volunteered to work on *Arthritis Today*'s 2005 and 2006 *Drug Guides* and this project:

Steven Abramson, MD
Daniel Clauw, MD
Doyt L. Conn, MD
N. Lawrence Edwards, MD
Don L. Goldenberg, MD
Eric L. Matteson, MD
Larry W. Moreland, MD
Harold Paulus, MD
Kenneth Saag, MD
Lee Simon, MD
Frederick Vivino, MD

Foreword

The number of people living with arthritis and other musculoskeletal disorders is vast, currently 66 million in the U.S. alone. That number is expected to increase substantially over the coming decade. The daily challenges of arthritis – pain, fatigue, stiffness and other symptoms – profoundly affect quality of life. Fortunately, there is a growing array of newly developed prescription drugs and widely available over-the-counter (OTC) medications that effectively treat these symptoms and, in some instance actually prevent permanent damage to joints and reduce the risk of disability.

This book – *The Essential Guide to Arthritis Medications* – was developed by the Arthritis Foundation and *Arthritis Today* magazine to provide up-to-date, unbiased information on nearly 250 name-brand and generic drugs approved for treatment of osteoarthritis, rheumatoid arthritis, fibromyalgia, lupus, gout, osteoporosis and other related conditions. Based on the yearly, award-winning *Arthritis Today Drug Guide,* this book's content has been thoroughly reviewed by an independent, volunteer panel of experts in the field of arthritis and related diseases.

It is our hope that the book will be a useful educational tool for people living with arthritis, and that this knowledge will help them better understand their treatment options, and more effectively work with their health-care professionals in order to lead a more active, fulfilling life with arthritis.

Medications are merely one part of a comprehensive self-management plan for people with arthritis, a plan that should also include proper diet, exercise, joint protection, and regular treatment by a physician. The Arthritis Foundation is dedicated to improving the lives of people with arthritis and related diseases through public health, public policy and research initiatives. Arthritis Foundation chapter and branch offices are located in communities across the nation, and these offices provide health information, community services and programs to help you live better with arthritis.

JOHN H. KLIPPEL, MD
President and CEO
Arthritis Foundation

*I*ntroduction

Ever since the ancient Greek healer Hippocrates used the leaves and bark of a willow tree to create a forerunner to our modern-day aspirin, people have probably used medications of one form or another to treat joint pain and related problems. While aspirin is still used more than 2,400 years after that early physician's experimentation with pain relievers, thousands of other drugs now join it in treating all that ails mankind.

As ever more drugs are developed and make it to market, medical consumers now have a dizzying array of options of treatments from which to choose. Making sense of all these choices is no easy task.

That's why the Arthritis Foundation decided to create this A-to-Z guide to arthritis medications. The book features an alphabetical, easy-to-read listing of the nearly 250 drugs most likely to be a part of your arthritis treatment plan, along with brand names, special instructions, side effects, precautions and more information for each drug. We hope you'll use it as a reference to learn about the medications you take now or one day may take for your arthritis.

The book also offers much more – basic information about the various classes of arthritis medications, why they're prescribed and the symptoms they relieve, as well as general advice to help you be better educated about the medicines you take, regardless of what those medications are.

When Hippocrates first gave his patients his willow-bark preparation, did they ask why he was giving them the drug? Did they ask its name, how long it would take to work, whether it caused side effects and, if so, which ones? Did they ask if it might interact with other drugs they were taking and if they should take it with food or on an empty stomach? Did they ask if there were other options besides willow bark if they didn't find it helpful? Did they learn all they could about the medication before they gave it a try? Who can say? If they didn't ask these questions, they probably should have. And so should you.

But how do you know what questions to ask? Making sense of medications today is far more complicated than just deciding how much bark to chew. We hope this book will help you open the lines of communication with your doctor, pharmacist or other health-care provider, to know the questions to ask and how and where to find the answers you need.

The more you know about your medications, the greater control you can take over your arthritis. By learning all you can about your drugs – as well as when and how to take them and what to watch for when you do – you can help your doctor help you receive the best care for your arthritis.

Chapter I

A Primer on Arthritis and Its Treatment

WHAT IS ARTHRITIS?

Literally translated, arthritis means joint (*arth-*) inflammation (*-itis*). But if you have it, or are close to someone who does, you're probably all too aware that it's often much more. Arthritis can also cause joint pain, stiffness and damage. It can greatly limit a person's quality of life.

For many forms of arthritis, joint pain and/or inflammation may be just part of the problem. That's because many types of the disease are systemic, meaning they can affect virtually any part of the body. Without effective treatment to stop the damaging inflammation, damage not only to the joints, but also to the skin, muscles, blood vessels and internal organs (including the heart, lungs and kidneys, and, in some cases even the brain) can occur.

More than 100 different medical conditions fall under the umbrella term of arthritis. These 100-plus conditions range from quite common to extremely rare. While joint involvement is the primary feature of some forms, for others, it may be just one part of a serious and even life-threatening disease process. Joint pain may also be a feature of diseases that are not arthritis or arthritis-related. For example, joint pain often goes along with leukemia (a type of cancer in which the body produces an abundance of abnormal white blood cells). But leukemia is *not* a common cause of joint pain and joint pain is not the primary feature of leukemia.

The vast majority of people who have arthritis have one or more of the most common forms of the disease or related conditions described here.

OSTEOARTHRITIS

The most common form of arthritis, osteoarthritis (OA) involves the wearing away of cartilage that normally cushions ends of the bones where they meet to form a joint. The most commonly affected joints are those of the knees, hips, fingers, neck and lower back. When OA affects the fingers, it can cause knobby bone growths (called nodes) that may be painful and interfere with the ability to enjoy leisure activities such as doing needlework, playing the piano or holding a golf club. OA, which affects an estimated 21 million Americans, becomes more common with increasing age.

RHEUMATOID ARTHRITIS

Rheumatoid arthritis (RA) is an inflammation of the synovium, the thin membrane that lines the joint, causing pain and inflammation. Sometimes inflammation is so severe that it damages cartilage, bone and connective tissue. The joints RA is most likely to affect are those of the fingers, hands, wrists, elbows, shoulders, knees, ankles and feet.

Although no one fully understands RA, it is generally believed to be an autoimmune disease in which the body's own immune system – which is designed to protect us from harmful invaders such as viruses and bacteria – mistakenly turns against healthy tissue. While the main sites of this attack are the joints, RA can affect you all over. You may run a low-grade fever, experience fatigue and have all-over achiness. In rare cases, RA can also affect the skin, muscles and internal organs, such as the heart and lungs.

BACK PAIN

Back pain is such a common problem that more than two-thirds of adults experience it at some point in their lives. The causes of back pain are varied. The most common cause is probably osteoarthritis. Other possible causes include injury from an accident or improper lifting, poor posture, pinched nerves, osteoporotic fractures, slipped or ruptured discs (the springy pads that provide cushioning between the individual bones of the spine, or vertebrae) or other forms of arthritis.

ANKYLOSING SPONDYLITIS

Ankylosing spondylitis is one of a group of diseases collectively referred to as the *spondyloarthropathies* (meaning arthritis that affects the spine) that typically affect the sacroiliac joints that attach the spine to the pelvis and the vertebrae that form the spinal column. In the most severe and advanced cases of ankylosing spondylitis, the tissues that support the spine can become ossified, or bonelike, causing the spine to stiffen and fuse in one position.

GOUT

One of the most acutely painful forms of arthritis, gout occurs when uric acid – a bodily waste product – builds up to such high levels in the blood that it seeps out and deposits as crystals in the body's tissues, including the joints. Gout usually strikes a single joint suddenly. Inflammation and swelling of the affected joint may be so severe that the skin over the joint is pulled taut and appears shiny and red or purplish. Typically, inflammation subsides on its own within a week or so, but unless the high level of uric acid is treated, attacks will return with increasing frequency and affect more joints, including the feet, knees and elbows. If allowed to progress, gout can lead to joint damage.

LUPUS

Systemic lupus erythematosus (SLE), often referred to simply as lupus, is an inflammatory disease that affects an estimated 250,000 Americans. It affects six times as many women as men and four times as many blacks as whites. It is most likely to begin during a woman's childbearing years. Like other forms of arthritis, lupus causes inflammation of the joints – typically those of the hands, wrists, elbows, knees and feet. But because it is a systemic disease, it can also affect the skin, blood, lungs, kidneys and cardiovascular and nervous systems, potentially leading to irreversible organ damage.

POLYMYALGIA RHEUMATICA

Although its name literally means pain in many muscles, polymyalgia rheumatica (PMR) is actually a joint disease. Inflammation in the joints of the neck, shoulders and hips causes stiffness and aching. PMR affects an estimated 450,000 people, and about 66 percent of those affected are women. The disease rarely occurs in people under 50; the average age at which PMR begins is about 70.

FIBROMYALGIA

Fibromyalgia is the most common arthritis-*related* condition, affecting some five million people – mostly women. It is characterized by widespread pain, fatigue that is often debilitating, and the presence of tender points, or precise areas on the body that are particularly painful upon application of the slightest pressure. Other problems commonly associated with fibromyalgia include sleep disorders; headaches; difficulties concentrating; frequent constipation or diarrhea, or a combination of the two, along with abdominal pain (a condition known as irritable bowel syndrome); bladder spasms or irritability or urgency (making you feel like you're always needing to go to the bathroom or that you have to go immediately); and pain in or problems with the temporomandibular joint (TMJ) that attaches the lower jaw to the skull on each side of the face.

OSTEOPOROSIS

The most common disorder of the bone, osteoporosis (or porous bones) is a condition in which the body loses so much bone mass that bones are susceptible to disabling fractures under the slightest trauma. The disease is most common in older women in whom the body no longer produces large levels of the bone-preserving hormone estrogen. In addition, some of the medications (namely, corticosteroids such as prednisone) used to treat inflammatory forms of arthritis can increase the risk of osteoporosis.

How Is Arthritis Treated?

An arthritis treatment plan usually has many different components. It may consist of a few or more of the following elements.

- Medications or drugs, both prescription and over the counter

- Physical therapy and exercise to improve the joints' range of motion, increase muscle strength and help relieve pain

- Bracing or splinting to stabilize affected joints

- Use of heat and cold to relieve pain and inflammation

- Occupational therapy to help you learn how to use joints more effectively with less stress

- Rest to allow the body and joints to recuperate between tasks

- Diet and weight loss to minimize the stress on joints due to excess body weight

- Water therapy to ease tightness of the connective tissues and relieve pain

- Surgery to replace damaged joints with prostheses or to stabilize joints

Regardless of the other components of their treatment plan, most people with arthritis require medications at some point. Although some drugs are used widely for many forms of arthritis, others are highly specific to the particular form of arthritis you have, its severity, and the symptoms you are experiencing.

WHAT IS A DRUG?

The Food and Drug Administration (FDA), the government agency that oversees and approves all drugs sold in the United States, defines drugs as "articles intended for use in the diagnosis, cure, mitigation, treatment, or prevention of disease in humans or other animals; and articles (other than food) intended to affect the structure or any function of the body of humans or other animals." One might further define a drug as a substance that is consumed orally, injected, inhaled, inserted, or applied topically and is absorbed into the body, as opposed to something that is placed in the body and remains essentially in its original form.

Although the definition states that drugs are intended to be useful for health, some people feel the word "drug" connotes illicit drug use and instead prefer to use the word "medication" to refer to drugs that are used legitimately for medical conditions. In this book, however, we'll use the words medication and drug interchangeably.

WHAT DO ARTHRITIS DRUGS TREAT?

Some arthritis medications are used primarily to ease symptoms (that is, to make you feel better), while others are used to slow or stop the underlying disease process. Many of them help symptoms *and* help slow or halt the disease process. Here are some of the specific problems arthritis medications are used to lessen, stop or even prevent:

- **Pain:** Most people with arthritis rate pain as their most troubling symptom, so it's not surprising that the most commonly used arthritis medications are those that ease pain.

- **Inflammation:** A normal immune system reaction to injury or infection, inflammation can also occur as the result of a faulty immune response in some forms of arthritis. The most common site of inflammation is the joints, which become red, hot, swollen and painful. In some forms of arthritis, inflammation can also occur in the skin and internal organs. Drugs to stop inflammation are among the most useful and widely used treatments for many forms of arthritis.

- **Joint damage/erosions:** Inflammation in the joint linings in RA can cause the bone to erode, or wear away, leading to joint instability and deformity. Some drugs that slow the disease process of RA have been proven to stop erosions and joint damage that are unfortunately common in the disease.

- **Other problems:** Depending on the particular form of arthritis or related condition you have, you may take medications to help with sleeping problems, low bone density, high blood levels of uric acid or other problems.

WHICH MEDICATIONS ARE USED IN ARTHRITIS TREATMENT?

Many drugs are used in arthritis and related conditions. In this book you'll learn about the most widely used medications for the most common forms of the disease. These medications, which we will discuss in Chapter 3 and which appear in the listing starting on page 55, fall into the following categories. (Keep in mind that depending on your specific condition your doctor may prescribe others.)

- Nonsteroidal anti-inflammatory drugs (NSAIDs)
- Cyclooxygenase-2 (COX-2)-specific inhibitors
- Salicylates
- Analgesics
- Topical analgesics
- Corticosteroids
- Disease-modifying antirheumatic drugs (DMARDs)
- Biologic response modifiers (BRMs)
- Fibromyalgia medications
- Gout medications
- Osteoporosis medications
- Sjögren's syndrome medications

Some categories of drugs – including NSAIDs, analgesics and corticosteroids – are used in almost all forms of arthritis. DMARDs – and increasingly the biologic response modifiers – may be used in a number of different diseases. Still others, such as those we will list under gout, Sjögren's syndrome medications, and osteoporosis medications, are fairly specific to those diseases. Fibromyalgia medications vary widely and include drugs used for other problems, including analgesics, muscle relaxants, antidepressants and sleep aids.

In addition to the drugs used for arthritis, we'll discuss some treatments that aren't technically drugs, but may seem like drugs. They include:

- Viscosupplements (or hyaluronic acid substitutes)
- *Prosorba* column therapy

Chapter II

Taking Medications:
What You Need to Know

At the first signs of joint pain, you may visit your local pharmacy (or simply look in your bathroom medicine cabinet) and select an over-the-counter (OTC) pain reliever. For some people with mild OA, for example, an occasional dose of OTC medication is sufficient. If pain persists or you notice other symptoms, however, you should see a doctor, who may prescribe different or stronger medications, other treatments to relieve symptoms and perhaps control the disease.

WHAT'S THE DIFFERENCE BETWEEN PRESCRIPTION AND OTC DRUGS?

Essentially the difference between an OTC and prescription medication is that you must have a doctor's written order – or phone call to the pharmacy – to receive a prescription drug. For OTC drugs, you need nothing but the money to pay for them. But that doesn't mean OTC drugs aren't serious medications.

When it comes to arthritis medications, the two types you'll find over the counter are the analgesic medication acetaminophen (*Tylenol*) and four nonsteroidal anti-inflammatory drugs (NSAIDs) – ibuprofen (*Advil, Motrin*), naproxen sodium (*Aleve*), ketoprofen (*Orudis KT*) and aspirin (*Bayer, Bufferin*). Although these drugs come in many formulations and in combinations with other ingredients (such as caffeine to speed pain relief, antihistamines to cause drowsiness, or a diuretic to ease menstrual bloating), these are the only over-the-counter medications you'll find to ease pain. These drugs often come in generic "store brands" as well.

Increasingly, drugs that were once available only by prescription are becoming available over the counter, a trend that has both benefits and drawbacks. On the positive side, getting a medication has never been more convenient and less expensive. You don't need an appointment with a physician if all you need is something to ease the pain of an occasional headache or muscle strain.

On the negative side, people are more likely than ever to self-medicate, not realizing they have a condition that requires the care of a physician. People also tend to think that anything they get over the counter is safe and that they can adjust the dosage as they see fit. This is not true. Even if you are taking an OTC medication, it's important to follow the directions exactly. You also should contact your doctor promptly if you suspect an adverse reaction or if symptoms don't improve.

It's also important to understand that OTC medications may be similar or identical to the ones prescribed by your doctor. Therefore, taking an OTC medication along with your prescription may lead to an overdose. Tell your doctor about *all* the medications you are taking at any time, including OTC medicines.

Fortunately, most OTC medications have new labels that will help people understand what's in them as well as how to take them. OTC medications that don't have the labels yet will be required by law to have them shortly. For more information, see "The New Medication Labels: What to Look For – and Heed" on page 20.

The New Medication Labels: What to Look For – and Heed

Similar to the Nutrition Facts that started showing up on food products a decade ago, all nonprescription medications now have a standard, easy-to-read label format. The Food and Drug Administration, which has mandated the new labels, is requiring minimum type sizes and other graphic elements to ensure the labels' readability.

The new labels will help you better understand what you are buying and easily find the information you need to take the drug safely. When reading any OTC medication label, it's important to pay careful attention to the following:

Dose – Find out how much you need and how often you should take it. (For children, doses of OTC drugs are usually given for both weight and age ranges. But it's best to go by a child's weight, if you know it.) If you're taking or giving a medication in liquid form, use a measuring spoon or measuring device from the pharmacy. The spoons included in most flatware sets probably aren't the right size, or they vary greatly in size. Stick with the dosage given on the label – unless your doctor advises otherwise. Never assume it's OK to take more medicine than the label says because you bought it over the counter.

Active ingredients – Look for words like acetylsalicylic acid, ibuprofen or acetaminophen. These are other names for aspirin, *Motrin* and *Tylenol*, respectively. If you're taking one of these drugs and then add another drug that contains one of them, you'll be setting yourself up for a potentially dangerous overdose.

Warnings – Whether it says to always take the medication with food or to avoid certain other drugs while on the medication, heed the warnings to minimize your risk of dangerous side effects or interactions.

Inactive ingredients – These are the ingredients that hold a pill together and give it its color and texture. Some people have allergies to the inactive ingredients, such as corn or food dyes. If you have any food allergies, be sure to check the inactive ingredients before taking a medication.

WHAT YOU SHOULD KNOW ABOUT YOUR MEDICATIONS

To make the most of your treatment program, gaining the most benefits with the least risk, it's important to know as much as you can about the medications you are taking – why they are used, the benefits you should expect from them and any adverse effects you should be aware of.

Before starting a new medication, you should ask your doctor the following questions:

- What is the name of the medication?
- How is this medication expected to help me?
- How long will I need to take it?

- Are there any special instructions for taking this drug?

- How long should I expect to wait before noticing effects?

- What should I do if I don't notice any benefit?

- Are there side effects I should be aware of?

- What should I do if I experience side effects?

- What should I do if I miss a dose of this medication?

- Is there anything I should avoid – certain foods, drinks, other medications, using heavy machinery, etc. – while using this medication?

- Is a generic available?

- If not, or if the medication is expensive, is there something similar that is less expensive?

- Is there anything else I should know about this medication?

Your pharmacist can also answer many of these questions concerning your medications, as well as whether your insurance will help pay for them and, if so, how much.

When getting a prescription filled, confirm the name of the drug with your pharmacist and why your doctor prescribed it. Because drug names can be similar – and doctors' handwriting is notoriously difficult to read – this will help guard against getting the wrong drug.

Once you have begun taking a drug, continue to ask questions. If you are concerned about how to take a drug or about a possible side effect or interaction you might be experiencing (see "How to Deal with Side Effects and

Interactions," page 24), call your doctor or other health-care professional. One plus to consulting a pharmacist is that they are usually available to answer your questions quickly.

What to Tell Your Doctor

Communication with your doctor is not a one-way street. Of course, there are questions you will want to ask, but there is also information your doctor will need from you. Here are some issues you need to bring up with your doctor before you begin a new medication.

• **Other medications you use.** Because medications have the potential to interact with one another (see page 26), it's essential that your doctor knows everything – including OTC drugs and nutritional supplements – you are already taking.

• **Diet restrictions.** Some medications have inactive ingredients that may not mesh with your dietary restrictions. If you have problems with alcohol, it's important to understand that many liquid medications contain alcohol.

• **Pregnancy and breastfeeding.** Because some medications can affect unborn babies and many others can be passed through the breast milk, it's important to let your doctor know if you are pregnant (or may become pregnant) or if you are breastfeeding.

• **Allergies.** If you have had allergic reactions to drugs – or even foods – let your doctor know. Even the inactive ingredients can trigger harmful reactions in some people.

> **What to Tell Your Doctor (cont.)**
>
> • **Other medical problems.** Some medical problems influence your body's ability to process certain drugs or increase your risk of a dangerous reaction. Let your doctor know about any medical problems you have and also problems that run in your family.

HOW TO DEAL WITH SIDE EFFECTS AND INTERACTIONS

Despite all the good they can do, all medications have their downsides. Two of these downsides are side effects and the potential for interactions.

SIDE EFFECTS

It is often said that anything strong enough to help is strong enough to cause harm. Any time you tamper with the body to solve one problem, you are likely to create another. The problem you create in the process is called an adverse reaction or a side effect.

Avoiding medication side effects isn't always possible. But there are things you and your doctor can do to minimize the risk. Here are a few:

• **Go low.** Your doctor will prescribe the lowest dose of medication that achieves the desired effects. While you should always take as much medication as you're prescribed (skipping doses or taking smaller doses on days you feel better can be dangerous), you should never take more medication than prescribed.

- **Follow directions.** Follow the medication's directions exactly. For example, taking a medication with food, for example, will make it less likely to irritate your stomach or cause nausea. Taking it at the proper time of day will ensure evenly spaced doses and reduce the risk of getting too much medication in your system at once.

- **Communicate with your doctor.** Let him know about any medical conditions you have in addition to the one he is treating. Sometimes, certain medical problems, such as kidney disease or ulcers, for example, may increase the likelihood of side effects from some medications.

- **Know the possibilities.** Become familiar with some of the most common side effects of the medications you are taking and ask your doctor what to do if you experience them. Some side effects may necessitate stopping a drug, some may resolve with time, and still others may be minor and tolerable compared to the problems you would experience from stopping an otherwise helpful drug.

- **Practice prevention.** Some side effects are so common that they can almost be anticipated. Others can be predicted because you've experienced them before. In cases like those, your doctor may prescribe another medication to help ease or prevent the side effect. For example, if you always get an upset stomach after taking an NSAID, your doctor may prescribe a stomach-protective medication along with your NSAID. If strong immunosuppressive drugs nauseate you, your doctor may prescribe an anti-nausea medication to be taken when it's time for your dose. Taking a folic acid supplement can prevent many of the side effects of methotrexate.

Medication side effects can run the gamut from minor annoyances that may (or may not) simply go away on their own to serious reactions requiring emergency attention. How to you know where your side effects rank along the continuum? The best advice is to ask your doctor ahead of time what to watch for – and then follow your instincts.

Side effects – and their urgency – vary largely by drug, so it's impossible to say what constitutes a serious side effect for each drug. For example, if you are using calcitonin nasal spray and you begin to have a runny nose or upper respiratory symptoms, it's probably nothing serious. You can take it easy, treat your symptoms with OTC products, if necessary, and call your doctor in a few days if you're not feeling a lot better. On the other hand, if you are taking a strong immunosuppressive drug such as azathioprine (*Imuran*), upper respiratory symptoms, such as a runny or stuffy nose or sore throat, could signal an infection that your suppressed immune system will have trouble fighting. Call your doctor right away.

For most side effects, a call to your doctor or pharmacist is sufficient. If, however, you experience severe bleeding, tightness in your chest, difficulty breathing, wheezing or hivelike swellings on your face and lips, don't stop to call your doctor. Call 911 or get to the closest emergency room immediately.

INTERACTIONS

In addition to causing adverse reactions individually, drugs may interact with one another to cause unwanted effects. In other words, two or more drugs that work well for you individually may not work as well or may even become dangerous when combined. (For a chart listing drugs that are likely to interact, see page 31.) These drugs' interactions, as they are called, fall into one of the following two categories:

- **Pharmacodynamic interactions.** These occur when one drug affects the absorption or elimination of another drug. When absorption is a problem, you won't get the full benefit of one drug you are taking because another drug is blocking it, making it less efficient. Thus a problem that was once controlled by a certain medication may go out of control. If elimination is a problem, you could end up with too much of a drug in your system, which could increase your risk of side effects from that drug.

- **Pharmacokinetic interactions.** These occur when two drugs with similar effects mix and essentially produce an overdose. For example, both aspirin and the blood-thinning drug warfarin (*Coumadin*) decrease your blood's ability to clot. If you are taking warfarin for cardiovascular disease and add aspirin to ease arthritis pain, you could be unwittingly setting yourself up for a life threatening bleeding episode.

To minimize your risk of drug interactions, it's important to let your doctor know every drug you are taking before you start a new one. That way, if possible, he or she can avoid prescribing drugs with the potential to interact. Following are some more steps you and/or your doctor can take to reduce the risk of harmful interactions:

- **Look beyond prescription drugs.** Prescription and OTC drugs aren't the only ones that interact with one another. Nutritional supplements also have the potential to interact with some drugs, as does alcohol (a common offender) and even some foods. When speaking with your doctor, don't forget to mention if you use nutritional supplements or alcohol. Also ask if there are any foods you should avoid while taking a medication.

- **Choose one doctor to coordinate your care.** If you see several different doctors for several different health problems, each may prescribe drugs not knowing what the others are prescribing. By having one doctor coordinate your care, you can minimize the risk of interactions among drugs prescribed by different doctors.

- **Write down everything you take.** Keep a thorough written record of what OTC and prescription drugs you take, the names of the doctors who prescribed them if they are prescription drugs, and at what dosage you take them. Also keep a record of what supplements you use, and write down the manufacturer of the supplement and the dosage you take. Take this written record to your medical appointments.

- **Pare down.** If you're taking many medications or you've been taking a prescription drug for so long that you can't even remember what it's for, find out from your doctor whether you still need to take all of your medications. There's a chance you don't or that there are newer, safer alternatives to one or more of the drugs you're taking.

- **Stick with one pharmacy.** Choose one pharmacy to fill your prescriptions and stay with it. Most pharmacies have computer programs that alert the pharmacist if another prescription you had filled at that pharmacy has the potential to react with your newest prescription.

- **Brown bag it.** Once a year fill a bag with all of the medications you are taking and have your pharmacist check them. The bag will contain the information – names of drugs and their dosages – that your pharmacist needs to determine if drug interactions are likely.

- **Adjust the timing.** Some medications interfere with others by keeping them from being them absorbed in the intestine. For example, antacids can interfere with the body's absorption of tetracycline and some other antibiotics. In those cases, your doctor may adjust the timing a bit – advising you to take one drug an hour or two after the other – to alleviate the problem.

- **Change the dosage – or the drug.** Sometimes two drugs interact to increase or decrease the effectiveness of one another. If a drug increases the effect of another, lowering the dose of one may help. In other cases, your doctor can switch you to a different drug that provides the benefits of the original drug without the interaction risk. (Note: you should never change your dosage on your own – speak to your doctor.)

- **Have regular monitoring.** If it's necessary for you to take two or more drugs that have the potential to interact, your doctor will need to monitor you closely, usually through frequent, regular blood tests. Unless a problem is actually detected, the risk of taking you off a medication – or perhaps even changing the dosage – may be worse than the risk of interactions.

- **Add another medication.** Although this is usually the choice of last resort, doctors must sometimes prescribe a third medication to help alleviate the problems that an interaction between two other drugs is causing. For example, if you need both NSAIDs and corticosteroids, yet taking them together causes stomach upset or increases your risk of developing a stomach ulcer, your doctor may prescribe a third drug such as cimetidine (*Tagamet*) or omeprazole (*Prilosec*) to ease your stomach upset and reduce your ulcer risk.

- **Be mindful of potential interactions.** Finally, if two drugs you are taking have the potential to interact, ask your doctor what symptoms you should watch for. Keep in mind that interactions aren't always immediate, nor are they always evident. But knowing what to watch for can help ensure you get medical attention (including a dosage or medication change) if you need it.

Drugs Likely to Interact

Many drugs people take for arthritis can interact with drugs they may take for other medical conditions. Following are some of the most commonly prescribed drugs and classes of drugs for arthritis and related conditions – and some of the drugs known to interact with them.

In some cases, you shouldn't take these drugs together. In others, your doctor may need to adjust the dosage or timing, or monitor you more closely for interactions. Remember, this is a just a sample of drugs that may interact. There is no way to list all of the possible combinations. You should always consult your doctor before taking one of these combinations, but also let your doctor or pharmacist know about all of the drugs you are taking before starting another:

Drug: NSAIDs
May interact with...
Corticosteroids; blood thinners such as warfarin (*Coumadin*); diuretic medications; antihypertensives (high blood pressure medicine); lithium; methotrexate; cyclosporine; other NSAIDs

Drug: Aspirin and other salicylates
May interact with...
Probenecid (*Benemid, Probalan*)

Drugs Likely to Interact (cont.)

Drug: Narcotic analgesics
May interact with...
The antiseizure medication carbamazepine (*Tegretol*); naltrexone, a drug taken for alcohol or drug dependence; tricyclic antidepressants such as amitriptyline (*Elavil*) or doxepin (*Adapin*)

Drug: Corticosteroids
May interact with...
Insulin or oral diabetes medications, such as metformin (*Glucophage*); antacids; growth hormones, such as somatrem (*Protropin*) or somatropin (*Genotropin*); diuretics; carbamazepine (*Tegretol*); phenytoin (*Dilantin*) and primidone (*Mysoline*)

Drug: Methotrexate
May interact with...
Aspirin or other salicylate medications; penicillin; probenecid; sulfonomides, such as sulfamethoxazole and phenazopyridine (*Azo Gantanol*), and sulfamethoxazole and trimethoprim (*Bactrim, Septra*)

Drug: Gold preparations such as auranofin
May interact with...
Penicillamine (*Cuprimine*)

Drug: Azathioprine (*Imuran*)
May interact with...
Allopurinol (for gout); other immunosuppressive drugs

Drug: Cyclophosphamide (*Cytoxan*)
May interact with...
Probenecid (*Benemid*) or sulfinpyrazone (*Anturane*) (for gout); antithyroid medications; antifungal medications or antiviral medications

Drug: Cyclosporine (*Neoral*)
May interact with...
Hormonal medications (including estrogens and androgens); allopurinol (*Zyloprim*) (for gout); cimetidine (*Tagamet*) (for ulcers); psoriasis medications; amiloride (*Midamor*); triamterene (*Dyrenium*)

Drug: Sulfasalazine
May interact with...
Acetaminophen (*Tylenol*); male or female hormones; lovastatin (*Mevacor*) and pravastatin (*Pravachol*) (for high cholesterol); carbamazepine (*Tegretol*) (for seizures); oral diabetes medications; blood-thinning medications

Drug: Alendronate (*Fosamax*)
May interact with...
Aspirin or aspirin-containing products

Drug: Estrogen medications
May interact with...
Acetaminophen (*Tylenol*); antithyroid medications; antimalarial drugs; divalproex (*Depakote*) and valproic acid (*Depakene*) (for seizures); cyclosporine; protease inhibitors such as ritonavir (*Norvir*)

Drugs Likely to Interact (cont.)

Drug: Raloxifene hydrochloride
May interact with...
Cholestyramine (*Questran*) (for high cholesterol); warfarin (*Coumadin*)

Drug: Teriparatide (*Forteo*)
May interact with...
Furosemide (*Lasix*)

Drug: Tricyclic antidepressant medications such as amitryptiline *(Elavil)* or doxepin (*Adapin*)
May interact with...
Amphetamines; appetite suppressants; asthma medications; cold medications; antithyroid medications; ulcer medications; monoamine oxidase (MAO) inhibitors

Drug: Selective serotonin reuptake inhibitors (SSRIs); including fluoxetine (*Prozac*) and sertraline (*Zoloft*)
May interact with...
Other antidepressants; the antihistamine astemizole (*Hismanal*); monoamine oxidase (MAO) inhibitors

Drug: Zolpidem (*Ambien*)
May interact with...
Monoamine oxidase (MAO) inhibitors

Drug: Temazepam (*Restoril*)
May interact with...
Other benzodiazepines

Drug: Benzodiazepines
May interact with...
Fluvoxamine (*Luvox*); itraconazole (*Sporanox*); ketocona-
zole (*Nizoral)* or nefazodone (*Serzone*)

Drug: Zaleplon (*Sonata)*
May interact with...
Carbamazepine (*Tegretol*); phenytoin (*Dilantin*); primidone (*Mysoline*); cimetidine (*Tagamet*) (for ulcers); central
nervous system depressants; tricyclic antidepressants

Drug: Cyclobenzaprine (*Flexeril*)
May interact with...
Other central nervous system depressants; monoamine
oxidase (MAO) inhibitors

Drug: Gabapentin (*Neurontin*)
May interact with...
Antacids such as *Maalox*

Drug: Allopurinol (*Lopurin, Zyloprim*)
May interact with...
Blood-thinning medications such as warfarin; immunosuppressive drugs such as azathioprine (*Imuran*) or mer-
captopurine (*Purinethol*)

Drug: Colchicine
May interact with...
Immunosuppressive drugs such as cyclophosphamide
(*Cytoxan*), azathioprine (*Imuran*) or methotrexate

Drugs Likely to Interact (cont.)

Drug: Probenecid (*Benemid, Probalan*)
May interact with...
Aspirin or other salicylate medications; cancer drugs; NSAIDs; blood-thinning drugs such as heparin

Drug: Sulfinpyrazone (*Anturane*)
May interact with...
Blood-thinning drugs such as heparin, or other sulfa-containing drugs such as celecoxib (*Celebrex*), sulfasalazine (*Azulfidine*) or sulfamethoxazole (*Bactrim*)

TAKING, TOSSING, REMEMBERING YOUR MEDICATIONS AND MORE

To get the most benefit from your medication, you know you need to take it exactly as prescribed. While the label will give you the basics, it may leave you with questions, such as "What time should I take my medications?" or "What should I take them with?" The following should help clarify some of the instructions on your prescription label.

WHEN IT SAYS TAKE WITH FOOD

Your prescription label says, "take with food." Does that mean you should only take your medicine at mealtime? Not necessarily. But you do need to eat *something* with your medication. A few crackers or a slice of bread usually will suffice.

In most cases, what you eat with your medication isn't important. However, there are some foods you should avoid when taking a particular medication. For example, eating foods rich in vitamin K (broccoli, cauliflower or brussels sprouts) may reduce the effectiveness of blood thinners prescribed to prevent clots after surgery. Likewise, consuming dairy products with tetracycline antibiotics and certain antifungals can reduce those drugs' effectiveness.

The prescription label or package insert you get from the pharmacy should let you know if there are certain foods you should avoid. If it doesn't, check with your doctor or pharmacist to be sure.

WHEN IT SAYS TAKE WITH WATER

If the label says to take the medication with water, wouldn't coffee, soda or juice work just as well? Maybe, but you'd be better off sticking with water. In some cases, your choice of beverages can have a serious effect on your medication.

Two beverages that have the potential to cause problems with medications are grapefruit juice and coffee. Grapefruit juice can cause blood levels of some drugs to rise to dangerously high levels. Drugs affected by grapefruit juice include the disease-modifying antirheumatic drug cyclosporine as well as antihistamines, anti-anxiety medications and cholesterol-lowering medications.

Research has shown that coffee can interfere with the effectiveness of the arthritis medication methotrexate. The caffeine in coffee – and to a lesser extent in tea and many soft drinks – is also known to lessen the effects of anti-anxiety medications and cause stomach irritation in people taking histamine (or H2) blockers for heartburn and stomach upset. It may also cause excessive central nervous system stimulation when taken with oral asthma medications.

A couple of exceptions to the water-only rule are NSAIDs and corticosteroids. Both of these can be taken with milk to reduce their risk of stomach irritation. (But don't make the mistake of taking other medications with milk, because milk may decrease the effectiveness of some medications, including certain antibiotics and antifungals.)

When taking your medication with water, be sure to drink the full eight-ounce glass and not just enough to wash it down. That will help ensure medicine doesn't linger in and irritate your throat.

WHEN IT SAYS TAKE ON AN EMPTY STOMACH

Some medications work best when taken on an empty stomach. So when is your stomach empty? Typically two hours after you have eaten and 30 minutes before you eat anything else.

WHEN IT SAYS TAKE
ONCE/TWICE OR MORE A DAY

The label on your prescription bottle will tell you how many times a day you need to take your medication, but most labels won't tell you exactly *when* to take your medication. Does timing matter? In many cases, the precise time you take a medication isn't important. What *is* important is that you take your medication regularly.

Because most medications work best when they remain at constant levels in your bloodstream, you should strive to space your doses evenly. For example, if you take a drug once a day, take it at the same time each day. If you take it twice a day, space your doses 12 hours apart. Three daily doses should be spaced eight hours apart and so on. Of course, there are some exceptions. Some osteoporosis drugs should be taken first thing in the morning, as should single daily doses of corticosteroids.

Experimenting with the timing of a single daily NSAID dose may help you get relief when you need it most. If you have any questions about when to take a medication, you should ask your doctor or pharmacist.

WHAT IF I CAN'T SWALLOW PILLS?

While the vast majority of arthritis medications come in the form of a tablet, capsule or caplet, not all do. And, often the drugs that come in pill form also come in – or can be made into – another form.

Here are some examples:

- Some corticosteroids and DMARDs, including methotrexate, come in injectable form as well as pill form. At least one oral corticosteroid, prednisolone sodium phosphate (*Pediapred*) is available as a liquid for easy swallowing.

- Acetaminophen and some NSAIDs come in the form of a rectal suppository.

- Some NSAIDs, including ibuprofen (*Motrin*), come in an oral suspension (liquid) form as well as tablets or capsules.

- Estrogen can be administered by a patch as well as a pill.

If you need to take a medication that comes only in a pill form, there are still a few things you and/or your pharmacist can do to make your pill more palatable. Here are some examples:

- **Crush it.** Crush the pill's contents and mix them with food, such as a spoonful of chunky peanut butter or a cup of applesauce. For some tips to see if your medication is crushable or can be crushed safely, see "Crushing and Splitting Pills," page 45, or speak with your doctor or pharmacist.

- **Coat it.** Ask your pharmacist if he or she carries empty gelatin capsules. If you have trouble swallowing chalky pills, your pharmacist may be able to crush them and place the contents into the capsules, which for most people slide down more easily than tablets.

- **Transform it.** If you can't find a form of medication you can take easily, consult a compounding pharmacist. These specialty pharmacists, who specialize in tailor-made medications, may be able to turn your prescription into a more palatable form, such as a flavored liquid, chewable tablet or even a popsicle! To find a compounding pharmacist near you, contact the International Academy of Compounding Pharmacists at (800) 927-4227 or search by zip code on their Web site, www.iacprx.org.

WHERE AND HOW DO I STORE MEDICATIONS?

Ironically, the two places many people store their medications — in a damp bathroom medicine cabinet or sunny kitchen window sill – are among the worst possible places. Exposure to direct sunlight or humidity can decrease the effectiveness of medication.

The best place to store your medication so that it retains its potency is away from heat, light and moisture, so dresser drawers and closet shelves are good bets. Unfortunately, out of sight can mean out of mind, and if you aren't in your closet or looking through your drawers frequently, you just might forget to take your medications. If that happens, your kitchen counter or other highly visible location (away from direct sunlight) would be a better option.

It's best to store your medications in the containers they came in from the pharmacy. That's because many medicine containers are amber-tinted to block out damaging light. If arthritis in your hands makes it difficult to open child-resistant containers, have someone remove the tops and place them lightly back on the bottle for easy removal. One word of caution: If you have small children in the house and aren't able to use child-resistant bottles, you'll have to lock up your medications and find tricks for remembering to take them. (For some suggestions that may help, see page 43.)

Some medications have special storage needs – for example, biologic response modifiers and some antibiotics must be kept in the refrigerator. Any special storage instructions should be on the medication's label. If you're in doubt about the proper way to store a medication, be sure to ask your pharmacist.

WHEN MEDICATIONS EXPIRE

You're halfway through a bottle of pills when you notice the expiration date – a week ago last Thursday. What do you do with the rest of the pills: take them or toss them?

If the expired medication hasn't hurt you yet, chances are you can continue to take it another week or two without any ill effects. But the medication may not be as potent – and therefore not as useful – as when it was newer. If you need a medication to control a disease process, that in itself can be dangerous.

In some cases an expired medication can be harmful in a more direct way. Aspirin and the antibiotic tetracycline, for example, can break down and their breakdown products can be toxic to the kidneys.

Perhaps more important than the age of the medication is the condition of the medication. Medication that is not stored properly (see how to store medications, page 40) may lose its potency even before the expiration date. If you open a medication bottle and notice the pills look different or have an odd smell, that means they are deteriorating – throw them away immediately, regardless of the expiration date.

Some liquid medications will have a "beyond use" date, which is calculated from the time the drug was mixed at the pharmacy and printed on the drug's label. You should always throw away a drug when it reaches the "beyond use" date.

If you're ever in doubt about a medication, your best choice is to throw it out. Though discarding medication may seem like an expensive waste, taking a medication that fails to control your disease or causes kidney damage can be far more costly. Contact your doctor's office if you have to throw out a medication and may need a new prescription.

HOW TO DISPOSE OF MEDICATIONS

When it comes time to discard old medications, experts discourage throwing them in the trash where they may be retrieved and consumed by someone. Flushing your medications down the toilet is easy and will keep them from being found and ingested, but doing so has the potential to contaminate the water supply. The safest way to dispose of drugs, if you're so inclined, is to place them in a container and return them to your pharmacy or physician's office for safe, environmentally friendly disposal.

---

10 Tips for Remembering to Take Your Meds

For a medication to work, you have to take it. If you find yourself forgetting a dose now and then, the following tips may help you remember:

1. If you take a medicine twice a day, place it next to your toothbrush and take it when you brush in the morning and at bedtime.

2. If you take a medication in the morning, place it next to your coffee pot, your toaster or your cereal box where you'll be certain to see it first thing.

3. If you take a medicine just before going to bed, place it on your nightstand, next to your lamp or alarm clock.

---

10 Tips for Remembering to Take Your Meds (cont.)

4. To remember medications all day long, post reminder notes on your refrigerator, microwave oven, computer screen, bathroom mirror or steering wheel – anywhere you'll see them often.

5. Use a container with days-of-the-week compartments available at most pharmacies. Some are divided for different medications and/for several daily doses. Fill the container every Sunday evening for the coming week.

6. Keep your medications where you are – in your purse, your pocket, your briefcase or desk drawer. When it's time to take them, you will have them close at hand; plus seeing them every time you open your drawer or purse will serve as a constant reminder. One word of caution: avoid leaving medications in the car, where they may get too hot on a warm, sunny day and lose their effectiveness.

7. Keep a daily listing of medications and the times you are scheduled to take them. Keep the calendar in a central location, perhaps your kitchen, or electronically on your computer calendar if you use one. Check off each medication as you take it.

8. Set your wristwatch to ring an alarm when it's time to take your medication.

9. Take your medications at the same time every day and eventually it will become a habit.

10. Let family members know the medications you are taking and when you need to take them – ask them to remind

you. One note: while this two-heads-are-better-than-one approach can be helpful, remember that you are the one ultimately responsible for remembering your medicine.

While it's important to do all you can to remember your medications, it's also important to acknowledge that sometimes you're bound to slip up and miss a dose. Find out now from your doctor or pharmacist what you should do in the event that that happens. Generally you should take the missed dose of medication if not much time has passed since you were supposed to take the dose. On the other hand, if it's almost time for the next dose, just skip the missed dose and take the next dose at its regularly scheduled time. But it's best to ask your doctor.

CRUSHING AND SPLITTING PILLS

Suppose your doctor has prescribed one 50-mg dose of a drug daily, but your pharmacy carries only 100-mg pills. Would it be OK to get the larger strength pills and divide them? Or suppose the new capsules you're taking are so large they make you gag. Would it be OK to crush them and mix them with a glass of water?

The answer depends on the medication in question. In some cases, it's OK to split or crush a pill; in other cases it's not. If you are uncertain as to whether a particular pill or capsule can be safely split or crushed, it's always best to ask your pharmacist. However, the following page lists some general guidelines for when it's all right and how to go about it.

- **Look for a line.** If a tablet is scored – that is, it has a grooved line running down the center – it's OK to split. If a tablet is not scored, it's still probably OK to cut it but you will need a pill cutter, available for about $4 to $5 in most drugstores.

- **Do the crush test.** Most tablets that can be cut are also safe to crush. To determine if a tablet is safe to crush, place it in a plastic bag and then try crushing it with the back of a spoon. If the tablet crushes easily, it's probably OK to take. If it doesn't, toss it and take your remaining tablets whole.

- **Check its coat.** In general, any tablet that has a gel coating should not be split or crushed.

- **Try to open it.** If a capsule opens easily, it's probably OK to open it and mix the contents with water (as long as you drink all of the mixture immediately). If a capsule is sealed, it should probably stay that way.

- **Check the timing.** Pills or capsules that are formulated to release a drug into your bloodstream slowly through-out the day should never be split or crushed. Medications for arthritis that fall into this category include *Voltaren, Voltaren-XR, Arthrotec, Lodine, Lodine XL, Indocin SR, Relafen, Naprelan* and *EC-Naprosyn*. If you are not sure whether a medication you have been prescribed is time-released, speak to your doctor or pharmacist before opening, breaking or crushing it.

PAYING FOR DRUGS

If you have arthritis – particularly if you take drugs for it regularly or if you have other conditions in addition to arthritis – drugs may take a large chunk out of your monthly income, even if you have good health insurance. For some lower-income people – or those without health insurance – drug costs can easily *exceed* income. Whether you're paying a lot for your drugs or can't afford to take the drugs your doctor prescribes, there are options to reduce your costs and/or get access to the drugs you need. The following suggestions should help.

Understand your drug coverage. Find out from your insurer or employer's benefits manager exactly what your insurance policy covers. For example, does it cover a brand-name drug when a generic version is available? (See "Opt for generics," page 48) Does it cover generics at a higher rate than brand-name drugs? Are there drugs your policy won't cover? When at all possible, guide your doctor to prescribe drugs that are covered by your insurance. If you need a drug that isn't covered, find out what your recourse is – sometimes special documentation from your doctor will do the job. For specific questions you should ask your insurer or employer, see page 53.

Ask for samples. Don't spend a lot of money for a drug until you know if it works. Doctors routinely receive samples of drugs from the manufacturers' sales reps. If your doctor prescribes a drug that you may have to use for a long time, ask if he or she has any samples. You may be able to use them while you wait to see how the drug works for you or while you wait to see if you qualify for some type of assistance with your medication costs. (See "Find out what Medicaid and Medicare offer" and "Go to the manufacturer," both on page 50.)

Opt for generics. If given a choice between a brand-name drug and a generic, opt for the generic. The generic is almost always cheaper. Here's why: When a company develops a new drug, it applies for a patent, which prohibits anyone else from marketing the drug for 20 years. This time of exclusivity allows the company to recoup the costs of developing and testing the drug, which averages about $360 million per medication. After the patent has expired, other manufacturers may duplicate and market their own versions of the drug, called generics. Because makers of generic drugs don't have to repeat the extensive clinical trials to prove the safety and efficacy of their drugs, their expenses are much less and they can pass those savings along to you.

Patent issues aside, generic and brand-name drugs are essentially same. You may notice differences in packaging and minor differences in taste and appearance, but the medication inside – the reason you are taking the drug – is the same whether you get the generic or brand-name product.

Check into mail-order pharmacies. If you take medications regularly over a long period of time you may get them for a lot less by mail order than you could from you neighborhood pharmacy. For example, with one health plan we investigated, the copayment for a 30-day supply of a generic drug from a local pharmacy was $10, while the copayment of a 90-day supply (an additional 60 days' worth) was just $15. In addition to cost savings, mail-order pharmacies offer convenience. If you fill out the paperwork and get a doctor's prescription once, they will send your medications every 90 days – no repeat trips to the pharmacy, waiting for prescriptions to be filled, or hassle of keeping up with it all – for you. See the box on this page to find out how to contact some of the major mail-order pharmacies.

Mail-Order Pharmacies

If you have insurance coverage, check to see if your insurer works with a particular mail-order pharmacy. If not, here are some you might want to try.

Caremark
(800) 966-5772 / www.caremark.com

Chronimed Bioscrip
(specializes in injectable medications)
(800) 801-8886 / www.bioscrip.com

TRICARE Mail Order Pharmacy (for military personnel)
(866) 363- 8667 / www.tricare.osd.mil/pharmacy/tmop.cfm

Express Scripts
www.express-scripts.com

Find out what Medicaid and Medicare offer. As of 2006, prescription drug benefits subsidized by the government that provide some type of assistance to older and disabled citizens who are unable to pay for their medications fall under Medicare Part D. If you are disabled from arthritis or another medical condition or if you are over age 65, this is an option worth investigating. Depending upon the specifics of your eligibility you may be able to get drugs at significantly reduced rates. To find out if you qualify for additional drug assistance, log onto www.medicare.gov or contact your state Medicare program. You can get your State Health Insurance Assistance phone number from the Medicare helpline at (800) 633-4227. The Kaiser Family Foundation at www.kff.org is another good source of information.

Go to the manufacturer. Most drug manufacturers have patient assistance programs that offer free or discounted drugs to people who are unable to pay for them. Contact the manufacturer of the drug you are interested in learning if it offers such a program. While you can make the initial contact, in most cases your doctor will need to fill out the paperwork necessary to get the medication.

The Pharmaceutical Research and Manufacturers of America (PhRMA) offers a directory of programs that provide drugs to physicians whose patients cannot otherwise afford them. For a copy of the directory, call (800) 762-4636 or log onto www.pparx.org. If you don't qualify for a patient assistance program, contact the manufacturer to see if it offers a pharmacy card. If you meet certain income requirements, you can purchase a card for a nominal charge (and, in some cases, they're free) that can be used to get a discount on medications from selected pharmacies. Many manufacturers offer their own pharmacy cards. Others manufacturers offer cards jointly. Together RX, for example, is a prescription drug program that offers discounts of 20 to 40 percent on more than 155 medications from several manufacturers. To find out more, log onto www.togetherrx.com

Check with organizations. If you are a member of an organization, check and see if it offers special discounts on prescription drugs for members. If you are a member of AARP, you may be eligible to receive a 17 percent discount on brand-name drugs and about 50 percent off on generics. You can search the AARP drug database to find your medications and then order directly from the association.

If you are in the military or a retired veteran, you can get prescription drug coverage through the Veteran's Administration. TRICARE is the regionally managed health-care program for active duty and retired members of the uniformed services, their families and survivors. For more information, visit one of the following Web sites: www.tricare.osd.mil or www.tricare-online.com or call toll-free (866) 363-2273.

Check with your pharmacy. Many drugstore chains offer discounts to seniors or discount cards to all frequent shoppers. Check to see what perks pharmacies in your area offer.

Shop online. You can buy just about anything online these days and drugs are certainly no exception. In fact, if you have an e-mail address, your inbox may be filled with ads from online pharmacies offering discounts on the medications you want and need without the inconvenience of seeing a doctor.

While you can possibly save between 10 and 30 percent on drugs by ordering them online, be sure to do so with a prescription from your *own* doctor. Despite what some sites would have you believe, it's important to get your prescriptions from a doctor who knows you and your medical history – not an unknown entity who has you answer some questions via computer.

When choosing an online pharmacy, look for one with a VIPPS (Verified Internet Pharmacy Practice Sites) seal indicating approval from the national Association of Boards of Pharmacy. Also do some price comparisons – both with other online sites and your own local pharmacy – to be sure you're getting a bargain. Also, find out any costs you'll incur in addition to the cost of the medication itself. Shipping, handling and other fees can quickly negate any savings.

Consider special circumstances. If you have a rare form of arthritis, you may be eligible for financial assistance with your drugs from organizations that help people with rare diseases, such as the National Organization for Rare Disorders. If you don't qualify for other assistance programs, this is a possibility worth pursuing. You'll find the National Organization for Rare Disorders online at www.rarediseases.org.

Exhaust all your options. If you know you must qualify for some assistance but haven't been able to find it, check out the Benefits Check Up established by the National Council on Aging. It can help you identify your eligibility for a variety of assistance programs. You'll find the program online at www.benefitscheckup.org.

Questions to Ask Your Insurer or Your Employer

If you have insurance, it's important to know what your policy will cover – and how much it will pay – before you fill your prescription. Here are some questions to ask your insurer or employer's benefits manager about your drug coverage:

- Where can I find a list of covered drugs? (Or, is the drug I need covered?)

- If the plan doesn't cover my drug, does it cover a comparable one? (For example, if the plan doesn't cover the specific NSAID your doctor prescribes, does it cover a selection of other NSAIDs that might work for you?)

- What should I do if my doctor feels I need a drug that is not on my formulary? How can I petition to have it covered?

- How much does the plan pay for brand-name drugs?

- How much does it pay for generics?

- Is the plan only good at selected pharmacies?

- Can I save money on medications by using preferred pharmacies?

- Can I save money by purchasing a 90-day supply versus a 30-day supply?

Chapter III

Drugs to Treat Arthritis and Related Conditions

As we discussed in Chapter 1, medications are almost always part of an arthritis treatment plan. Depending on the form of arthritis or related condition you have and the specific complications associated with it, you may take medications to ease pain, relieve inflammation, stop or prevent internal organ damage, strengthen bones, relax aching muscles, lessen flares, promote sleep or slow, stop or even prevent joint damage.

In this chapter, we'll discuss some of the specific types of medications used in the treatment of arthritis and related conditions. Some of the medications we'll discuss are used for many different conditions, whereas others are unique to a particular disease.

Here are some of the types of medications that may be part of your treatment plan.

NONSTEROIDAL ANTI-INFLAMMATORY DRUGS (NSAIDs)

Regardless of the type of arthritis you have, you have probably taken one or more drugs from a class called nonsteroidal anti-inflammatory drugs (NSAIDs). Considered first-line agents (the first drugs a doctor prescribes before moving on to stronger drugs, if necessary), NSAIDs are often effective at relieving pain and inflammation – two major problems for people with arthritis.

The largest class of drugs used for arthritis, NSAIDs include one of the oldest and most widely used medications – aspirin – as well as the popular over-the-counter medications ibuprofen (*Advil, Motrin IB, Nuprin*), ketoprofen

(*Actron, Orudis KT*) and naproxen sodium (*Aleve*), which are available in higher doses by prescription. About a dozen other NSAIDs are available only by prescription.

All NSAIDs ease pain and inflammation by blocking the production of chemicals in the body called prostaglandins, which also play a role in numerous other bodily functions, including blood clotting, menstrual cramps, labor contractions, kidney function and stomach protection. Recent studies on a handful of NSAIDs suggest these drugs may increase the risk of heart attack or stroke. For that reason, it's important to discuss with your doctor any history of heart disease or cardiovascular risk factors before you begin taking an NSAID.

Also, because blocking the stomach protective prostaglandins puts NSAID users at risk of gastric bleeding and ulcers, you should always be watchful for symptoms of stomach ulcers – vomiting blood, frank red blood in stools or black, tarry stools. If you notice symptoms or if you're not sure, stop taking the NSAID and call your doctors.

In recent years, a subclass of NSAIDs was developed to be safer for the stomach. This subclass, called COX-2 inhibitors, work by selectively inhibiting cyclooxygenase-2 (COX-2), the enzyme that is responsible for the production of inflammatory prostaglandins involved in arthritis, without interfering with COX-1, a similar enzyme that is responsible for the production of prostaglandins that protect the stomach. At one time, three COX-2 inhibitors were on the market. Two were withdrawn after studies showed increased risk of cardiovascular events. Other possible risks included gastric bleeding and severe skin reactions. As of the time this book was printed, celecoxib (*Celebrex*) was the only COX-2 inhibitor on the market.

If you have a history or ulcers or risk factors for them (see "Ulcer Risk Factors," page 59), your doctor may prescribe celecoxib instead of a traditional NSAID. Other factors that will help determine which NSAID you will take include the following:

- **Your doctors' familiarity with the drugs.** Because there are so many different NSAIDs, most doctors select four or five different ones and then prescribe one of those for all patients.

- **What works best for you.** Some people seem to do better on certain NSAIDs than others. If your first – or second or third – NSAID doesn't significantly improve pain and inflammation, your doctor may try another drug or a different pain-management approach.

- **Convenience.** If you prefer the convenience of taking just one pill a day, you may want an NSAID that comes in an extended release formulation, instead of one that must be taken two or three times a day. Be aware, however, that one-a-day medications are not the best option for all people. Because they stay in the body longer than drugs designed to be taken more frequently, they may not be safe if your body has trouble metabolizing drugs or if other factors put you at increased risk of side effects.

- **Cost.** Some NSAIDs (particularly the ones that are available as generics) cost considerably less than others, and some insurance companies may cover only certain NSAIDs. When all other factors are equal or similar, you may prefer the most affordable NSAID option.

Ulcer Risk Factors

Your risk of suffering an NSAID-related stomach ulcers increases if you:

• Are older than 65

• Have had stomach ulcers or GI bleeding in the past

• Use corticosteroids along with NSAIDs

• Use high doses of NSAIDs or more than one NSAID at a time

• Use NSAIDs over a long period of time

In addition, you may be at increased risk of stomach ulcers if you:

• Smoke

• Drink alcohol

• Have a *helicobacter pylori* infection

• Have more than one health problem

WHEN NSAIDs UPSET YOUR STOMACH

Any time you take a medication for one problem, you risk experiencing another. For the millions of Americans who use NSAIDs, that other problem often involves the stomach. Because traditional NSAIDs inhibit the body's production of prostaglandins, hormone-like substances that protect the stomach lining, using these drugs can lead to problems ranging from occasional nausea and heartburn to bleeding ulcers.

Fortunately, there are ways to minimize your risk of these problems. While the most notable is using a COX-2 inhibitor, that's only one possible solution. Here are three other options:

- **Using safer meds.** Another subclass of NSAIDs, called nonacetylated salicylates, are chemically related to aspirin but formulated to be easier on the stomach than aspirin or other traditional salicylates. Nonacetylated salicylates include such drugs as choline and magnesium salicylates (*CMT*, *Tricosal*, *Trilisate*), choline salicylate (*Arthropan*), and magnesium salicylate (*Magan*, *Mobidin*, *Mobogesic*), among others.

  Other types of NSAIDs that might be easier on the stomach include buffered tablets, enteric-coated tablets that don't dissolve until they reach the small intestine, and time-released capsules or tablets that release the drug slowly into the bloodstream.

- **Replacing prostaglandins.** By replacing the stomach's natural protective prostaglandins, a synthetic prosta-glandin product called misoprostol (*Cytotec*) – when used along with NSAIDs – can reduce the risk of new ulcers or promote the healing of existing ulcers. One product, marketed under the name *Arthrotec*, combines the NSAID diclofenac sodium with misoprostol.

- **Blocking stomach acid.** If you have a problem with NSAID-related indigestion, heartburn or nausea, you may benefit from taking a drug that reduces the amount of acid produced by your stomach. These drugs, which can be taken along with your NSAID, come from two categories, histamine blockers (or H2 blockers) and proton pump inhibitors. Histamine blockers include such drugs as cimetidine (*Tagamet*), rantidine hyrdrochloride (*Zantac*), famotidine (*Pepcid*) and nizatidine (*Axid Pulvules*). Proton pump inhibitors include omeprazole (*Prilosec*) and lansoprozole (*Prevacid*). (It's important to note that neither proton pump inhibitors nor H2 blockers decrease the risk of GI bleeding.)

Although several acid-blocking drugs are available over the counter, you should always check with your doctor before taking one of them along with NSAIDs. And remember, despite all of the safer NSAIDs and medications available to ease NSAID-associated stomach problems, all NSAIDs do carry some risk of stomach problems.

ANALGESICS

If your arthritis is painful – and it's the rare case of arthritis that isn't – you may find relief from an analgesic, or pain-reliever. Analgesic medications are used purely for pain relief. They don't work on inflammation or other disease symptoms that other arthritis medications do.

The most commonly used and readily available analgesic is acetaminophen (*Tylenol*). Based on its cost, effectiveness and safety, the American College of Rheumatology recommends acetaminophen as a first line of treatment against osteoarthritis pain. For many people, acetaminophen alone is sufficient to ease OA pain.

Acetaminophen can be purchased over the counter under a variety of different trade and store names and is often the active ingredient in products labeled "aspirin-free pain reliever."

Until recently, acetaminophen was virtually the only analgesic medication used for day-to-day arthritis pain. Although doctors sometimes prescribed much stronger narcotic analgesics such as oxycodone (*OxyContin, Roxicodone*) or propoxyphene hydrochloride (*Darvon, PP-Cap*) for their arthritis patients, these types of pain relievers have traditionally been used for the acute pain of surgery, osteoporotic fracture or severe musculoskeletal pain.

The thinking has been that these drugs, when used for more than short-term, acute pain, can lead to physical and psychological dependence. People may need larger and larger doses to provide the same amount of pain relief and grow dependent on the drugs psychologically as well. However, years of experience have failed to show that, when used appropriately, these drugs present a high risk of dependence. Furthermore, the medical profession as a whole now focuses on the importance of treating nonmalignant pain and the unique ability of narcotics to ease pain. In fact, when the American College of Rheumatology revised its guidelines for treating osteoarthritis in 2000, it acknowledged for the first time the role of narcotic analgesics in treating osteoarthritis pain. One analgesic, tramadol (*Ultram*), was mentioned specifically in the group's treatment guidelines.

Because analgesic medications don't influence prostaglandin production the way NSAIDs do, they don't carry NSAIDs' risk of ulcers. But they do have side effects of their own, which may include drowsiness, grogginess, constipation and the potential for dependence.

TOPICAL ANALGESICS

If you have just a few painful joints or if oral analgesics or NSAIDs fail to sufficiently control your pain, an option worth trying is a topical analgesic. Topical means that you apply the medication (usually a cream or salve) directly on the skin where the pain is located. In fact, the American College of Rheumatology's treatment guidelines for OA of the hip and knee acknowledge the role of topical analgesics for OA pain, particularly in people whose pain is mild to moderate and not relieved by acetaminophen alone.

These topical creams, salves and rubs are available OTC under various brand and store names. They work using one or more of these active ingredients:

- **Counterirritants.** Like stepping on your toe to take your mind off a headache, counterirritants stimulate or irritate the nerve endings to distract the brain's attention from musculoskeletal pain. Counterirritants encompass such substances as menthol, oil of wintergreen, camphor, eucalyptus oil, turpentine oil, dihydrochloride and methlnicotinate and are found in products such as *ArthriCare*, *Eucalyptamint*, *Icy Hot* and *Therapeutic Mineral Ice*.

- **Capsaicin.** A highly purified natural ingredient found in cayenne peppers, capsaicin works by depleting the amount of a neurotransmitter called substance P that is believed to send pain messages to the brain. For the first couple of weeks of use, the ingredient may cause burning or stinging. Capsaicin is available under the product names *Zostrix*, *Zostrix-HP*, *Capzasin-P* and others. *Menthacin* includes both capsaicin and counterirritants.

• **Salicylates.** Like the salicylates found in many oral pain relievers, these compounds may work by inhibiting prostaglandins. They primarily work topically as counter-irritants, themselves stimulating or irritating nerve endings. Brand-name examples of topical analgesics containing salicylates include *Aspercreme*, *Ben-Gay*, *Flexall*, *Mobisyl* and *Sportscreme*.

Unlike most other arthritis medications, which are swallowed or injected, these rubs work on the area into which you rub them, minimizing the risk of systemic side effects.

CORTICOSTEROIDS

Potent inflammation-fighting drugs, corticosteroids are used in virtually all diseases characterized by inflammation, including many forms of arthritis. In diseases such as rheumatoid arthritis, lupus, polymyalgia rheumatica, polymyositis and giant cell arteritis, corticosteroids work quickly to stop inflammation that threatens the joints, kidneys, blood vessels or other organs.

The most-prescribed corticosteroid for arthritis-related diseases is oral prednisone (*Deltasone, Orasone, Prednicen-M, Sterapred*). It is one of the least expensive drugs you could take for arthritis, costing just pennies a day. There are also several other corticosteroids, including cortisone acetate (*Cortone*), prednisolone (*Prelone*) and methylprednisolone (*Medrol*).

Although most people with arthritis take corticosteroids daily by mouth, if you have severe organ-damaging inflammation, your doctor may administer high doses intravenously (IV) over the course of a few days. If you have just one or a few inflamed joints, your doctor may inject a corticosteroid compound directly into the affected joint(s) for quick, temporary relief without wide-ranging side effects. If you have psoriasis or an arthritis-related skin rash, you doctor may prescribe a corticosteroid ointment.

Particularly when used in high doses and/or long term, corticosteroids are associated with a number of side effects, including Cushing's syndrome (weight gain, moon face, thin skin, muscle weakness, brittle bones), cataracts, hypertension, increased appetite, elevated blood sugar, indigestion, insomnia, mood changes, nervousness or restlessness. Minimize those risks by using the lowest doses that keep your disease under control.

Some doctors reduce the risk of corticosteroid side effects by prescribing alternate-day therapy (that is, you take your dose every other day, instead of every day). But this practice is controversial. Other doctors feel that only daily doses of corticosteroids can effectively control inflammation.

DISEASE-MODIFYING ANTIRHEUMATIC DRUGS (DMARDs)

When nonsteroidal anti-inflammatory drugs – and, sometimes, low doses of corticosteroids – fail to control the pain and inflammation of arthritis, doctors prescribe disease-modifying antirheumatic drugs (DMARDs). As their name suggests, DMARDs actually modify the course of the disease, slowing or perhaps even preventing the disease process and its ensuing joint damage. Most rheumatoid arthritis patients will be placed on a DMARD in addition to NSAIDs and low doses of corticosteroids.

DMARDs are used in inflammatory forms of arthritis, such as rheumatoid arthritis, psoriatic arthritis and ankylosing spondylitis. Most of them work by suppressing the immune system, which is involved in the joint damage that occurs with these diseases. DMARDs are not effective against the more common osteoarthritis.

If your doctor prescribes a DMARD, be prepared to wait a while for results. Since most of these drugs take from several weeks to several months to work, your doctor may prescribe other drugs to help your symptoms while you wait for your DMARD to take effect. Once a DMARD is started, some people take them indefinitely; others have to change DMARDs periodically, when one starts to lose its effectiveness and something new is needed to control the disease. For others, however, DMARDs can bring on a remission of the disease – or a period of disease inactivity – during which they no longer need a DMARD to control their disease.

In 1998, a drug called leflunomide (*Arava*) became one of just a few DMARDs developed specifically for rheumatoid arthritis. Most DMARDs originally were used and approved for other medical conditions. Methotrexate, for example, was originally a cancer treatment. Cyclosporine (*Neoral*) and mycophenolate mofetil (*CellCept*) were used to prevent organ rejection in people who had undergone transplants, and hydroxychloroquine sulfate (*Plaquenil*) was used to treat malaria. It was only after years of use for these other conditions that they were approved or used for rheumatic diseases or that RA-specific brands were developed.

Despite the new drugs developed in recent years, the existing DMARDs continue to play an important role in managing rheumatoid arthritis. Methotrexate (*Rheumatrex, Trexall*), for example, is considered by many rheumatologists to be the "gold standard" for RA treatment. Even people who take one of the newer biologic agents (see Biologic Response Modifiers, below) often take methotrexate along with it. Other, older DMARDs, including oral and injectable gold, are rarely used any more.

Like all drugs, DMARDs are associated with side effects. (For specific side effects of the various DMARDs, see the A to Z listing starting on page 89.) With most, the most serious is an increased risk of infection. If you are taking any drug that suppresses your immune system and you begin to experience symptoms of an infection, such as a sore throat, fever or chills, you should call your doctor immediately.

BIOLOGIC RESPONSE MODIFIERS

Unlike older immunosuppressive drugs, which cause widespread suppression of the immune system, the biologic response modifiers (also referred to as biologic agents, or simply biologics) modify the immune system by targeting chemical messengers called cytokines that play a role in the inflammation and damage of the disease.

Five of the six currently available agents work by either blocking or inhibiting the production of inflammatory cytokines that are believed to play a role in the inflammation and destruction of RA and other diseases. Abatacept (*Orencia*), adalimumab (*Humira*), etanercept (*Enbrel*), and infliximab (*Remicade*) target a cytokine called tumor necrosis factor (TNF), while anakinra (*Kineret*) blocks a different cytokine, interleukin-1 (IL-1). The most recently approved biologic agent for RA, rituximab (*Rituxan*) works by blocking CD20+ B cells that have been shown to be key players in rheumatoid arthritis and some other diseases.

By blocking these cells and cytokines that are involved in the disease process, the biologic agents retard the inflammatory response and thus ease the signs and symptoms of RA – usually in people for whom nothing else had worked. But research has shown these drugs do more than make people feel better. They also help prevent joint damage. While some doctors reserve biologic agents for people whose arthritis hasn't responded to more conventional therapies, others are starting to prescribe them before exhausting other treatment options (a process that can take years) in an effort to prevent damage from the disease.

The downside of the biologic agents is that they must be injected. Etanercept, anakinra and adalimumab are injected through a small needle just beneath the skin. Infliximab, abatacept and rituximab are administered intravenously in a doctor's office or infusion center. Another downside is cost – a year's course of any of these drugs can cost $15,000 or more. Still another caveat is that because of the drugs' newness, it is impossible to predict if they will have any long-term side effects. Studies thus far, however, show the drugs are relatively safe.

For reasons probably related to differences in genetics or the specific disease process, some people respond better to one biologic than another. Sometimes a doctor will switch you from one biologic to another if the first doesn't produce sufficient results.

On the drug-approval horizon are biologics that may inhibit more than one chemical and biologics that can be taken orally.

OSTEOPOROSIS MEDICATIONS

Not so long ago, women who were past menopause and expressed concerns about the brittle-bone disease osteoporosis to their doctor were automatically handed a prescription for estrogen replacement therapy. That's because estrogen, a bone-preserving hormone, is lacking in women after menopause. Replacement hormones can help correct the deficit and keep bones strong – and for a time they were the only drugs available to do that. But unfortunately they were not without some potentially serious risks (including cancer), and the hormones weren't appropriate for men or for younger people – either male or female – with bone loss.

Although hormone replacement therapy is still used today, it is now just one of many treatment options for women who have or are at risk of developing osteoporotic fractures. Not only that, one of the newer drugs, alendronate (*Fosamax*) is approved for men and also used in children who are at risk of osteoporosis.

The best medication for you will depend on a number of

factors, including your sex, drug preference, other health problems you have or are at increased risk for, and whether you already have osteoporosis or are trying to prevent it.

Medications for osteoporosis prevention and/or treatment fall into the following general categories. Whichever treatment your doctor prescribes, ask about the advisability of taking calcium and vitamin D supplements, both of which enhance the body's natural bone-building or bone-preserving abilities.

ESTROGEN

Still often used for post-menopausal women is the female hormone estrogen (*Premarin, Estratab, Menest*). For women who have not had a hysterectomy, doctors prescribe estrogen in combination with the hormone progesterone (*Premphase, Prempro*) to minimize any risks of estrogen on the uterus. If you are going through menopause and experiencing troublesome hot flashes and other symptoms, estrogen replacement can ease those symptoms as well as prevent bone loss. But estrogen is not for every woman. If you have a history – or family history – of breast or uterine cancer, you may not be a candidate for hormone replacement. All women should speak with their doctors about the benefits and risks of this therapy.

CALCITONIN

Another hormone used to treat osteoporosis is calcitonin, which is similar to a hormone produce by our parathyroid glands (two pairs of endocrine glands that are situated behind or within the thyroid gland). Naturally occurring in the body, parathyroid hormone controls the distribution of calcium and phosphate in the body and has been shown to have an effect on bone growth. Calcitonin, which is administered as a nasal spray (*Miacalcin*), has been shown to reduce fracture risk. It also has some pain-relieving effects for people who have already had fractures.

BISPHOSPHONATES

A class of medication used in the treatment of bone diseases, including Paget's disease, bisphosphonates are being used increasingly in the treatment of osteoporosis as well, because they inhibit bone resorption. In recent years, two bisphosphonate medications (alendronate [*Fosamax*] and risedronate sodium [*Actonel*]) were approved for osteoporosis. Risedronate sodium is approved specifically for corticosteroid-induced osteoporosis. Unlike many of the other medications used for osteoporosis, bisphosphonates are appropriate for men.

SELECTIVE ESTROGEN RECEPTOR MOLECULES

One of the newest classes of medications for osteoporosis, selective estrogen receptor molecules (SERMs), including raloxifene hydrochloride (*Evista*), work much like estrogen to slow bone loss. The biggest difference: they lack some of estrogen's side effects, mainly those related to breast and uterine tissue, making them an attractive alternative to estrogen replacement for women at increased risk of breast or uterine cancer.

BONE FORMATION AGENTS

The newest class of drugs used in osteoporosis treatment is the bone formation agents. The first and only drug in the class thus far, teriparatide (*Forteo*), was approved in December 2002. Given by injection, the drug stimulates new bone formation and reduces fracture risk. Teriparatide is approved for the treatment of both men and women with osteoporosis who are at high risk of a fracture.

FIBROMYALGIA MEDICATIONS

If you have fibromyalgia, you likely use some of the drugs used for arthritis pain – namely NSAIDs or analgesics – to help relieve the muscle aches and possibly headaches associated with your condition. Your doctor may also prescribe some medications that aren't used in other forms of arthritis or related conditions.

Although no drugs are approved specifically for fibromyalgia, a number of medications have been proven to be effective for the condition in randomized clinical trials. These include the antidepressant medications, such as amitriptyline (*Endep*), duloxetine (*Cymbalta*), and fluoxetine (*Prozac*); muscle relaxants, such as cyclobenzaprine (*Cycloflex, Flexeril*); and certain analgesics, including tramadol (*Ultram*).

These and other drugs used in fibromyalgia work in a variety of different ways to ease the common problems characteristic of the condition.

If your doctor prescribes a medication for fibromyalgia,

be sure to let him know if you are taking any nutritional supplements, particularly ones like SAM-e and St. John's wort that are used for depression. By combining these with many of the antidepressants used in the treatment of fibromyalgia you may increase the side effects of the drugs.

Because there are so many different medications that can be used in fibromyalgia, we can't possibly discuss all of them in this book. We have included only those that have been tested in fibromyalgia. However, doctors have found success treating patients with other classes of medications, such as sleep medications, anti-anxiety medications and some anti-seizure medications.

ANTIDEPRESSANTS

When administered in smaller doses than those used to treat depression, antidepressant medications, including the tricyclics (amitriptyline hydrochloride [*Endep*], doxepin [*Adapin, Sinequan*] and nortriptyline [*Aventyl, Pamelor*]) and the selective serotonin reuptake inhibitors (SSRIs, such as fluoxetine [*Prozac*], paroxetine [*Paxil*] and sertraline [*Zoloft*]) may both help with mood disturbances and enable people with fibromyalgia get the deep, restorative sleep they need.

MUSCLE RELAXANTS

Muscle-relaxing medications, such as cyclobenzaprine (*Cycloflex, Flexeril*), may help reduce muscle spasms associated with fibromyalgia and also help induce deep sleep.

GOUT MEDICATIONS

Gout attacks can happen suddenly, causing severe pain. Fortunately, there are medications that can ease future attacks or prevent them altogether. In fact, gout is one of the most treatable forms of arthritis. To select the right medication for you, your doctor needs to determine the exact underlying problem.

Gout is caused when excess uric acid builds up in the body and is deposited as crystals in body tissues, including the joints and skin. If you have gout because your body produces too much uric acid, a drug called allopurinol (*Lopurin, Zyloprim*) will slow the rate of uric acid production and help prevent future attacks. On the other hand, if the build up is related to your body's inability to excrete uric acid properly, another drug – probenecid (*Benemid, Probalan*) – may help prevent attacks by increasing the amount of uric acid passed in the urine.

While preventing future attacks is certainly a goal for anyone with gout, the medications used to prevent gout attacks do little, if anything, to ease an attack once it has started. And ironically, any of these drugs may at first cause an increase in gout attacks as the body mobilizes uric acid. For that reason, your doctor should prescribe an NSAID or anti-inflammatory drug called colchicine along with these uric acid regulators to ease the pain and inflammation of resulting attacks.

Once an attack has started, NSAIDs or corticosteroids can provide symptomatic relief.

In addition to prescribing drugs for your gout, your doctor may also recommend you exercise, reduce weight, drink plenty of water, and limit alcohol and foods high in purines – organ meats, anchovies, sardines and fish roe – both of which are known to exacerbate gout.

WHEN ONE DRUG ISN'T ENOUGH

Even with the ever-increasing medication options for arthritis and related conditions, it's not likely you'll find a single drug that both relieves your symptoms and controls the underlying disease. In this case, your doctor may prescribe a combination of drugs.

Here are a few examples of common combinations:

- If you have rheumatoid arthritis, you may take an NSAID to help ease pain and inflammation and a DMARD (or perhaps more than one DMARD) to get your disease under control.

- If you take a biologic response modifier for RA, you may also need to take an NSAID and a DMARD.

- If you have lupus, you may take a DMARD, such as hydroxychloroquine sulfate (*Plaquenil*), to help control the disease, along with a corticosteroid to help prevent inflammation-related damage to internal organs such as the kidneys.

- If you have gout, you may take a drug like allopurinol (*Lopurin*, *Zyloprim*) or probenecid (*Benemid*, *Probalan*) to control levels of uric acid in your blood, but you may also need an anti-inflammatory drug, such as an NSAID, corticosteroid or colchicine, to control the pain and inflammation of gout attacks.

• If you take the biologic agent infliximab (*Remicade*), you will need to take methotrexate along with it. The addition of methotrexate not only adds to the effectiveness of *Remicade*, it helps prevent your body from forming antibodies to the drug.

• If you use a slow-acting drug such as hydroxychloroquine sulfate (*Plaquenil*) to treat rheumatoid arthritis or lupus, your doctor may prescribe another drug, such as an NSAID, to relieve symptoms while you wait for the *Plaquenil* to work.

• If you have fibromyalgia, you may need an analgesic to help relieve pain, a muscle relaxant to ease muscle spasms and a sleep aid to help you rest.

Increasingly doctors are learning that combining drugs may produce a synergistic effect. That is, two drugs together may provide benefits greater than one or both would produce alone. In some cases, drugs may be combined because one drug reduces the negative effects, or side effects, of another.

There are virtually unlimited combinations of drugs prescribed. The particular combination you will take, if you need it, will depend on your specific form of arthritis, its symptoms and severity, as well as your body's response to specific medications. Other health problems you have will also play a role in the drug combination you receive.

Keep in mind two cautions about drug combinations. Keeping up with which drug to take when can be difficult.

Make a daily list or calendar of drugs and the times to take them and follow it faithfully until you memorize it. (For more tips on remembering drugs, see page 43.) Also, you should always remember to keep up with the name of each medication you take and why you take it and to always be mindful of potential drug interactions.

MEDICATIONS FOR OTHER ARTHRITIS-RELATED PROBLEMS

If you have arthritis, there's a fair chance that arthritis isn't the only medical condition you have. Other problems can accompany arthritis, and some forms of the disease have associated problems that require treatment beyond that used for the arthritis itself. Following are some of the more common associated conditions and treatments for them:

Sjögren's syndrome. An autoimmune disease that affects the body's moisture-producing glands, Sjögren's syndrome can occur on its own or along with such diseases as RA or lupus. If dry eyes and mouth bother you, medical products available both over the counter and by prescription can help.

Two oral medications, pilocarpine hydrochloride (*Salagen Tablets*) and cevimeline hydrochloride (*Evoxac*) are approved for treating dry mouth associated with Sjögren's syndrome. Because both drugs can cause excessive sweating, it's important to drink plenty of water to avoid dehydration while using them.

For dry mouth that is less severe, artificial saliva products in the forms of rinses or sprays can help. Sample brands of such products include: *MouthKote, Optimoist, Oralbalance,*

Salivant and *Salivart*. Such products can also be used along with *Salagen* or *Evoxac* or to provide additional relief at times of particularly troublesome dryness, such as before bedtime or meals. These products are available without a prescription. If you don't find them on your drugstore's shelves, ask your pharmacist to order them.

For dry eyes of Sjögren's syndrome, doctors may prescribe cyclosporine ophthalmic emulsion, a specially formulated version of the immunosuppressive drug cyclosporine, to treat moisture-robbing inflammation.

Although they are not approved for such, both *Salagen* and *Evoxac* may also help ease dry eyes associated with Sjögren's syndrome. Artificial tear products, including *Bion Tears, Gonak, Isopto Tears, Lacril, Nature's Tears* and *Ocucoat,* can also ease dry and gritty-feeling eyes. Another product, hydroxypsopyl cellulose pellets (*Lacrisor*), when placed in the lower eyelid, can seal in the moisture provided by these eyedrops.

Psoriasis. For people with psoriatic arthritis, joint involvement is accompanied by scaly patches of skin known as psoriasis.

For many people with psoriatic arthritis, both the joint and skin problems are managed with disease-modifying drugs such as sulfasalazine (*Azulfidine*) or methotrexate; immunosuppressive drugs, such as azathioprine (*Imuran*) and cyclosporine (*Neoral*) or the biologic agents etanercept (*Enbrel*) and infliximab (*Remicade*).

If these treatments alone don't clear the skin problems, doctors may prescribe additional mediations for the skin.

These include the following:

- Steroid ointments and creams

- Topical coal tar preparations, such as *Tegrin* and *T-Gel*

- Calcipotriene (*Dovonex*) – a synthetic form of vitamin D3 applied topically

- Tazarotene (*Tazorac*) – a prescription retinoid (vitamin A) derivative applied topically

- Anthralin (*Drithocreme, Dritho-Scalp, Micanol*) – a prescription topical medication

- Salicylic acid – an over-the-counter topical preparation

More severe skin involvement may be treated by a systemic drug called psoralen along with exposure to ultraviolet-A light.

Irritable bowel syndrome. By some estimates as many as 70 percent of people with fibromyalgia have symptoms of irritable bowel syndrome (IBS), including abdominal pain and bloating, along with constipation or diarrhea or alternating bouts of the two.

Two drugs, alosetron hydrochloride (*Lotronex*) and tegaserod maleate (*Zelnorm*), are approved for irritable bowel syndrome. *Lotronex* is used to treat diarrhea-prominent IBS; *Zelnorm* is used to treat the multiple symptoms of abdominal pain, bloating and constipation.

Although *Zelnorm* and *Lotronex* are the only drugs approved for IBS, doctors may prescribe others. Among the most commonly used are from a class called anticholinergic (antispasmotic) drugs, which can reduce the overactivity of the intestine in people prone to IBS-related diarrhea. These drugs include dicyclomine (*Bentyl, Spasmoban*) and hyoscyamine (*Anaspaz, A-Spas S/L, Cytospaz, Donnamar, ED-Spaz, Gastrosed, Levbin, Levsin, Symax SL*).

Antiphospholipid antibody syndrome. People with the autoimmune condition antiphospholipid antibody syndrome, often seen in conjunction with lupus, develop antibodies to the lipid (fatty) membrane of cells and are at risk for potentially dangerous blood clots. To prevent clots in people with this condition, doctors may prescribe one of several medications. In some people, low-dose aspirin reduces clotting risk significantly; others require more potent anticoagulant medications, such as warfarin (*Coumadin*) or heparin (*Calciparine, Liquaemin*).

TREATMENTS THAT ONLY SEEM LIKE DRUGS

Along with the drugs on these pages, your doctor may prescribe some other therapies that may seem like drugs, but technically are not drugs. Here are two common ones:

HYALURONIC ACID SUBSTITUTES

For OA pain in the knee that isn't relieved by NSAIDs or analgesic medications, a relatively new class of products called hyaluronic acid substitutes or viscosupplements may help.

These products – hylan G-F 20 (*Synvisc*) and hyaluronate sodium (*Euflexxa, Hyalgan, Supartz, Orthovisc*) – are delivered directly into the knee through a course of three or five injections. Both products may relieve pain and are most effective for people with mild to moderate knee OA.

At first glance, the hyaluronic acid substitutes appear to be drugs. The FDA however, classifies them as medical devices. That's because instead of being absorbed into the body (a qualification for a "real" drug), these products are designed to supplement or replace hyaluronic acid, a substance that gives joint fluid its slippery quality and that appears to be low in people with arthritis. In that respect, the hyaluronic acid substitutes are more like a joint prosthesis than a pain-relieving medication, such as ibuprofen. They replace what is damaged; they are not designed to produce a pharmacologic effect in the body.

So far, the products are not approved for injection into joints other than the knee. It is not known whether they would provide the same pain-relieving effects when used in other joints.

PROSORBA COLUMN THERAPY

One approach to the treatment of rheumatoid arthritis, *Prosorba* column therapy uses a cylinder about the size of a soup can to filter disease-causing antibodies from the blood. During the *Prosorba* procedure, blood is removed through a vein in one arm, routed through the column and then returned through a vein in the opposite arm. The procedure typically takes place in a blood bank or a hospital's apheresis center. It is administered in 12 weekly sessions, each lasting two to two-and-a-half hours.

Though the process may seem similar to that used to infuse some intravenous drugs – including infliximab, (*Remicade*), cyclophosphamide (*Cytoxan*) or sometimes high doses of corticosteroids – *Prosorba* is not a drug. Nor does *Prosorba* column therapy involve administering a drug. Rather than infusing a substance *into* the body, the goal of *Prosorba* therapy is to mechanically filter and remove harmful antibodies *out* of the body. The *Prosorba* column is classified and regulated by the FDA as a medical device.

Prosorba column therapy is FDA-approved for people whose RA has not responded to disease-modifying antirheumatic drugs.

More Resources

As you move on to the A to Z listing section of this book, we feel confident you have learned important information you need to know about the medications you take – or may one day take – for your arthritis. But we hope you have gained a great deal more – knowledge that will help you become a better consumer of medications and of health care in general.

It's important to understand that the purpose of this book is not to give you medical advice – only your physician or other health-care provider can do that. What this book can do is serve as a starting point for establishing lines of communication with your health-care providers and playing a more active role in your health care. In today's fast-paced environment with ever-increasing treatment options, becoming your own health-care advocate is a must.

As you consider an arthritis treatment plan, research your options and discuss them with your physician. If there is a medication you want to know more about, don't wait for your doctor to make the first move. Come to your medical appointments armed with information and an attitude that together you can control your arthritis.

If your doctor prescribes one drug over another, find out why. If he or she prescribes an expensive medication, find out if there is a less expensive option. Find out which drugs your insurance company covers and what recourse you have if a drug you need isn't covered.

When you pick up any prescription, find out how to take it, what to watch for in terms of side effects and when – and which – side effects warrant a call to the doctor.

While only your doctor can prescribe a medication, remembering to take the medication and take it correctly is up to you. In other words, getting good results from any medication – and minimizing the less-than-good – is largely up to you.

The following sources can help you learn more about the medications you take as well as more general useful information on drugs:

AT THE LIBRARY OR BOOKSTORE

• *Physician's Desk Reference* (PDR) (Thomson Healthcare, 2006). Features up-to-date FDA-approved information on more than 4,000 prescription drugs and photos of the most prescribed drugs. To order, call (800) 232-7379 or visit the Medical Economics Web site at www.pdrbookstore.com

• *PDR for Nonprescription Drugs, Dietary Supplements and Herbs* (Thomson Healthcare, 2006). Contains full, detailed descriptions of the most commonly used nonprescription drugs and preparations, along with full-color photographs of hundreds of over-the-counter drugs for quick identification. To order, call (800) 232-7379 or visit www.pdrbookstore.com.

• *United States Pharmacopeia Dispensing Information (USP DI) Volume II Advice for the Patient, Drug Information in Lay Language* (Micromedex, 2006). Offers easy-to-understand information on more than 11,000 brand-name and generic medications marketed in the United States and Canada. To order, call (800) 232-7379 or visit www.pdrbookstore.com.

• *Complete Guide to Prescription & Nonprescription Drugs 2006* by H. Winter Griffith and Stephen Moore (Penguin Group, 2005)

• *How to Save Thousands on Prescription Medication* by Ira C. Robinson (Xlibris Corporation, 2003)

ON THE WEB

• **www.nlm.nih.gov/medlineplus/druginformation.html.** Offers information on thousands of prescription and OTC medications, provided through two drug resources – MedMaster, a product of the American Society of Health-System Pharmacists, and the *USP DI Advice for the Patient*, a product of the United States Pharmacopeia.

- **www.safemedication.com.** A Web site of the American Health-System Pharmacists, this site offers important information on using medications safely and wisely.
- **www.fda.gov.** The Web site of the Food and Drug Administration. Offers a search engine for looking up information about medications and numerous food- and drug-related subjects.
- **www.rxlist.com.** Offers a searchable database of information on thousands of drugs by brand or generic name.

Some medications, particularly the newer ones, have their own Web sites. For example, check out: www.forteo.com, www.synvisc.com, www.hyalgan.com, www.enbrel.com, www.rcmicade.com, www.kineret.com, www.humira.com, www.arava.com and www.celebrex.com.

OTHER IMPORTANT RESOURCES

The Arthritis Foundation. You'll learn more about arthritis medications in the Arthritis Foundation's bimonthly consumer magazine, *Arthritis Today*. Each year's January-February issue features the magazine's annual Drug Guide. To read *Arthritis Today*, check your local newsstand or call (800) 283-7800 to subscribe. To inquire about a specific brochure, contact your local Arthritis Foundation office or call (800) 568-4045. You also can search the Arthritis Foundation Web site for general information, to find other helpful books and videos, and to read selected *Arthritis Today* stories at www.arthritis.org.

Pharmacy handouts. Most pharmacies include a print-out with each prescription, telling you how to take the medication, and informing of you possible side effects and what to do if you experience them. Read and become familiar with it before starting your course of medication, and be sure to discuss any concerns with your doctor or pharmacist.

Package labels and inserts. Each medication, over-the-counter or prescription, comes from the manufacturer with a package insert detailing how the medication should be taken, who should and shouldn't take it, how it works and the side effects associated with it. Inserts can be found in over-the-counter medication packages. For most prescription medications you will never see the package insert unless you ask for it.

Your physician and pharmacist. If you have any questions about a medication, how it works or how to take, the best thing to do is ask.

The Essential Guide to

Arthritis Medications

*Prescription and Over-the-Counter
Treatments for Your Joint Pain from A to Z*

Throughout the A to Z section of this book, we have placed special symbols next to each entry to help you differentiate between them, recognize special use instructions, or to see what treatments are considered potentially dangerous in certain situations. Use this key to understand these symbols:

 May have possible interactions with drugs and/or alcohol

Take with water

Take with food or milk

Do not use if pregnant, breastfeeding or trying to conceive

This A to Z guide features nearly 250 of the drugs most commonly used in the treatment of arthritis and related conditions. The alphabetical listing should make it easy to find your medication, whether you know it by its generic or brand name. Drug information is written in a simple to read format.

Before you begin looking up your drugs, however, read the following important information to help ensure you find your medication and understand the data included about it.

HOW TO FIND A DRUG

The drugs in this guide are listed alphabetically. Both generic and brand names are included in the listing so you can find your drug whether you know it by a particular brand name or its generic name.

WHAT THE HEADINGS MEAN

Under each drug name, you'll find seven headings – brand name(s), type of medication, what it's used for, dosage, special instructions, possible side effects, be aware. Here's what you need to know about each heading:

Brand name(s): This is a listing of some of the most well-known brand names of each drug according to a panel of medical experts for *Arthritis Today*, whose names are listed in the acknowledgements section at the beginning of the book, as well as the *U.S. Pharmacopeia Dispensing Information: Advice for the Patient*. In cases where one brand is listed, it is usually the only brand. Where two or more are listed there may be others. The inclusion of a certain drug or brand does not imply endorsement by the Arthritis Foundation, nor does the exclusion of a drug or brand imply that it's inferior to those listed. Where applicable, brand names for both prescription and non-prescription versions of the drug are included.

Type of medication: Drugs used to treat arthritis and related conditions typically fall into one of several categories. You'll find information about each of the drug categories in this guide in Chapter 3. Some drugs come in both prescription and non-prescription (or OTC) brands; in these situations, the particular brand is identified as one or the other. If a drug is available over the counter, that will be noted; otherwise, the drug is only available by prescription.

What it's used for: The medications listed in this guide, in some cases, may be used for problems unrelated to arthritis. Here you'll find how the drug is used in arthritis treatment and/or for which arthritis related condition(s) it is used.

Dosage: Dosages of drugs may vary depending on the disease being treated. In this listing you'll see only the dosage range for arthritis or the disease specified in "What it's used for." Dosages listed are typically in milligrams (mg) or milliliters (mL) and range from the lowest to highest typically prescribed. In certain situations, some conditions require an initial high dosage of a medication followed by a lower maintenance-level dosage. For those conditions, we haven't included the initial high dosage in the range.

> Always follow medication packaging and your doctor's recommendations about the dosage level that's right for you and your particular situation.

In medicines that are available in both prescription and non-prescription or OTC brands, dosages will differ between the two, as the amount of medicine per dose in a prescription version of the drug is usually higher. In addition, some OTC brands of the same drug will have a higher amount of the active ingredient per dose than others; specific dosages are listed in those cases.

Also note that these dosages are for adults up to age 65. Older adults and children typically require lower dosages. Some of the drugs in this listing are not prescribed for children. Ask your physician or your child's physician for more information.

Special instructions: This gives you important information on when and how to take your medication. For example, if you need to take your medication with food or at bedtime, you'll find that information here.

Possible side effects: We have listed side effects identified as more common by our panel of medical experts.

Be aware: In this section, we've listed important considerations for you to think about while taking each drug, from special blood or eye tests you might need to any pre-existing conditions that might prevent you from taking the medication. Be sure to check to see if any of the cautions apply to you. If they do, discuss them with your doctor. He or she may change your dosage, monitor you for side effects or switch you to another drug.

Abatacept

Brand name (s):
Orencia

Type of medication: biologic response modifier

What it's used for: moderate to severe rheumatoid arthritis

Dosage: Dose is based on body weight and ranges from 500 mg to 1,000 mg per treatment for most people. After three initial infusions at 0, 2 and 4 weeks, infusions are repeated every 4 weeks.

Special instructions: Drug is given intravenously through a vein in the arm during a 30-minute infusion done in a doctor's office, clinic or hospital. Abatacept can be given along with disease-modifying antirheumatic drugs.

Possible side effects: cough; dizziness; headache; infusion reactions, including change in blood pressure, facial swelling, hives, trouble breathing; serious infections; sore throat

Be aware: Rheumatoid arthritis carries a higher risk of infection and lymphoma. It is uncertain whether this and other biologic response modifiers increase lymphoma risk. This agent should be discontinued if you have a serious or recurrent infection, exposure to tuberculosis or positive skin test for tuberculosis. Abatacept should be used with caution in patients with congestive heart failure (CHF).

Acetaminophen

Brand name(s):

Anacin (aspirin-free), Excedrin caplets, Panadol, Tylenol, Tylenol Arthritis Pain

Type of medication: Analgesic (OTC)

What it's used for: To relieve pain in any form of arthritis

Dosage: 325 to 1,000 mg every 4 to 6 hours as needed, no more than 4,000 mg per day (for all products except *Tylenol Arthritis Pain*); 1,300 mg every 8 hours as needed; no more than 3,900 mg in 24 hours (for *Tylenol Arthritis Pain*)

Special instructions: Do not use with any other product containing acetaminophen; do not use for more than 10 days for pain – unless directed by a doctor.

Possible side effects: When taken as directed, acetaminophen is usually not associated with side effects.

Be aware: If you consume 3 or more alcoholic drinks per day, consult your doctor before taking acetaminophen. Mixing acetaminophen with alcohol can cause liver damage.

Acetaminophen with Codeine

Brand name(s):
Phenaphen with Codeine, Tylenol with Codeine #3

Type of medication: Analgesic (narcotic)

What it's used for: Pain not relieved by plain acetaminophen

Dosage: 15 to 60 mg every 4 hours as needed

Special instructions: Never take more of this drug than your doctor prescribes because high doses of this drug can slow down breathing.

Possible side effects: Constipation, dizziness, lightheadedness, nausea, sedation, shortness of breath, vomiting

Be aware: If you consume 3 or more alcoholic drinks per day, consult your doctor before taking acetaminophen. This medication can cause liver damage. In case of an accidental overdose, contact a physician or poison control center immediately. Over time, this drug may cause psychological and physical dependence. Before taking this drug, let your doctor know if you use central nervous system depressants such as antihistamines (allergy medications), tranquilizers, sleeping medications, muscle relaxants or narcotic pain medication, or if you have one of the following: liver disease or history of alcohol or drug abuse. Avoid taking more than one product with acetaminophen.

Activella, see Estrogens

Actonel

Generic name:
Risedronate sodium

Type of medication: Bisphosphonate

What it's used for: Treatment or prevention of osteoporosis

Dosage: 5 mg per day in a single dose or 35 mg per week in a single dose

Special instructions: Take only with 1 cup of water first thing in the morning. Swallow pill whole while sitting or standing; stay upright; avoid food for 30 minutes.

Possible side effects: Abdominal or stomach pain, heartburn

Be aware: Before taking this medication, let your doctor know if you are taking aspirin or aspirin-containing products or if you have problems with the esophagus, stomach or kidneys. Blood levels of calcium and vitamin D must be normal before starting therapy.

Actonel with calcium

Generic name:
Risedronate with calcium

Type of medication: Bisphosphonate with calcium supplement

What it's used for: osteoporosis treatment and prevention

Dosage: Risedronate is taken in a single weekly dose of 35 mg; calcium tables taken other six days

Special instructions: Risedronate sodium: Take only with water in the morning. Swallow pill whole while sitting or standing; stay upright; avoid food for 30 minutes. Calcium tablets: Take with food.

Possible side effects: Abdominal or stomach pain; heartburn

Be aware: Before taking this medication, let your doctor know if you are taking aspirin or aspirin-containing products, or if you have problems with the esophagus, stomach or kidneys. Blood levels of calcium and vitamin D must be normal before starting therapy.

Actron

Generic name:
Ketoprofen

Other brand name(s):
Prescription: Orudis, Oruvail
Non-prescription: Orudis KT

Type of medication: NSAID (OTC)

What it's used for: To ease arthritis pain and inflammation

Dosage: 12.5 mg every 4 to 6 hours as needed

Special instructions: Do not take for more than 10 days for pain or more than three days for fever unless directed by a doctor. Do not take with other prescription or OTC NSAIDs. Take as directed at the same time(s) every day. If you experience stomach upset, take with food or a glass of milk or an antacid.

Possible side effects: Abdominal or stomach cramps, pain or discomfort; diarrhea; dizziness; drowsiness; edema (swelling of the feet); gastrointestinal bleeding; headache; heartburn or indigestion; nausea or vomiting; peptic ulcer

Be aware: Before taking this medication, let your doctor know if you drink alcohol or use blood thinners, or if you have or have had any of the following: sensitivity or allergy to aspirin or similar drugs, kidney or liver disease, heart disease, high blood pressure, asthma or stomach ulcers. Because stomach ulcers or internal bleeding can occur

without warning, regular checkups are important. Patients on long-term NSAIDs should have blood counts and liver enzymes checked periodically.

Unlike low-dose aspirin, there is little evidence that this or other NSAIDs will protect against heart attack or stroke. NSAIDs may be used with low-dose aspirin, but doing so may slightly increase your risk of gastric bleeding. Before taking this or any NSAID, tell your doctor if you take ACE inhibitors, lithium, warfarin or furosemide.

All NSAIDs may cause an increased risk of serious blood clots, heart attacks and stroke, which can be fatal. This risk may increase with dose and duration of use. Patients with cardiovascular disease or risk factors for cardiovascular disease may be at higher risk. These drugs should not be used for pain in people having coronary bypass surgery.

Adalimumab

Brand name(s):
Humira

Type of medication: Biologic response modifier

What it's used for: To ease RA symptoms, prevent joint damage and improve physical function in adults with moderately to severely active RA.

Dosage: 40 mg once every other week given by subcutaneous (beneath the skin) injection when given with methrotrexate. May be used alone or in combination with methotrexate or other DMARDs. Some patients not also taking methotrexate may benefit from taking 40 mg weekly.

Special instructions: Drug must be refrigerated but not frozen prior to use. Comes in prefilled syringes and may be injected into the thigh, abdomen or upper arm.

Possible side effects: Redness and pain, itching, swelling and/or bruising at the injection site; upper respiratory infection

Be aware: Rheumatoid arthritis carries a higher risk of infection and lymphoma. It is uncertain whether this and other biologic response modifiers increase lymphoma risk. This agent should be discontinued if you have a serious infection (such as pneumonia) or recurrent infections. Live vaccine should not be given along with this drug, but the flu vaccine or vaccine for pneumonia (*Pneumovax*) can be safely given.

Let your doctor know if you have a history of (or currently have) one of the following: active infection, recurrent infection, exposure to tuberculosis or positive skin test for tuberculosis; or if you have a nervous system disorder, including neurological disorders such as multiple sclerosis, seizure disorders, myelitis or optic neuritis.

Patients with congestive heart failure (CHF) should not be given this drug.

Advil

Generic name:
Ibuprofen

Other brand name(s):
Prescription: Motrin
Non-prescription: Motrin IB, Nuprin

Type of medication: NSAID (OTC)

What it's used for: To ease arthritis pain and inflammation

Dosage: 200 to 400 mg every 4 to 6 hours as needed; no more than 1,200 mg per day

Special instructions: Do not take for more than 10 days for pain or more than three days for fever unless directed by a doctor. Do not take with other prescription or OTC NSAIDs. Take as directed at the same time(s) every day. If stomach upset occurs, take with food, a glass of milk or an antacid.

Possible side effects: Abdominal or stomach cramps, pain or discomfort; diarrhea; dizziness; drowsiness; edema (swelling of the feet); gastrointestinal bleeding; headache; heartburn or indigestion; nausea or vomiting; peptic ulcer.

Be aware: Before taking this medication, let your doctor know if you drink alcohol or use blood thinners, or if you have or have had any of the following: sensitivity or allergy to aspirin or similar drugs, kidney or liver disease, heart disease, high blood pressure, asthma or stomach ulcers. Because stomach ulcers or internal bleeding can occur

without warning, regular checkups are important. Patients on long-term NSAIDs should have blood counts and liver enzymes checked periodically.

Unlike low-dose aspirin, there is little evidence that this drug or other NSAIDs will protect against heart attack or stroke. NSAIDs may be used with low-dose aspirin, but doing so may slightly increase your risk of gastric bleeding. Before taking this or any NSAID, tell your doctor if you take ACE inhibitors, lithium, warfarin or furosemide. Using ibuprofen along with low-dose aspirin may interfere with aspirin's effect in preventing heart attacks.

All NSAIDs may cause an increased risk of serious blood clots, heart attacks and stroke, which can be fatal. This risk may increase with dose and duration of use. Patients with cardiovascular disease or risk factors for cardiovascular disease may be at higher risk. These drugs should not be used for pain in people having coronary bypass surgery.

Alendronate

Brand name(s):
Fosamax

Type of medication: Bisphosphonate

What it's used for: To prevent or treat osteoporosis

Dosage: For corticosteroid-induced osteoporosis: 5 mg per day in a single dose (10 mg if postmenopausal); for general osteoporosis treatment: 10 mg per day in a single dose or 70 mg per week in a single dose; For osteoporosis prevention: 5 mg per day in a single dose or 35 mg per week in a single dose

Special instructions: Take with a full glass (8 ounces) of water first thing in the morning. Do not eat or drink anything else or take any other medication, including calcium tablets, for at least 30 minutes after taking the drug. Take medication while sitting or standing and stay upright for at least 30 minutes to avoid irritating the esophagus.

Possible side effects: Abdominal or stomach pain; heartburn

Be aware: Before taking this medication, let your doctor know if you have problems with the esophagus, stomach or kidneys. Blood levels of calcium and vitamin D must be normal before starting therapy.

Alendronate with vitamin D

Brand name(s):
Fosamax Plus D

Type of medication: Bisphosphonate with vitamin D supplement

What it's used for: To treat osteoporosis

Dosage: Single dose of 70 mg alendronate and 2,800 IUs vitamin D

Special instructions: Take with a full glass (8 ounces) of water first thing in the morning. Do not eat or drink anything else or take any other medication, including calcium tablets, for at least 30 minutes after taking the drug. Take medication while sitting or standing and stay upright for at least 30 minutes to avoid irritating the esophagus.

Possible side effects: Abdominal or stomach pain; heartburn

Be aware: Before taking this medication, let your doctor know if you have problems with the esophagus, stomach or kidneys. Blood levels of calcium and vitamin D must be normal before starting therapy.

Aleve

Generic name:
Naproxen sodium

Other brand name(s):
Prescription: Anaprox

Type of medication: NSAID (OTC)

What it's used for: To ease arthritis pain and inflammation

Dosage: 220 mg every 8 to 12 hours as needed

Special instructions: Do not take for more than 10 days for pain or more than three days for fever unless directed by a doctor. Do not take with other prescription or OTC NSAIDs. Take as directed at the same time(s) every day. If you experience stomach upset, take with food or a glass of milk.

Possible side effects: Abdominal or stomach cramps, pain or discomfort; diarrhea; dizziness; drowsiness; edema (swelling of the feet); gastrointestinal bleeding; headache; heartburn or indigestion; nausea or vomiting; peptic ulcer.

Be aware: Before taking this medication, let your doctor know if you drink alcohol or use blood thinners or if you have or have had any of the following: sensitivity or allergy to aspirin or similar drugs, kidney or liver disease, heart disease, high blood pressure, asthma or stomach ulcers. Because stomach ulcers or internal bleeding can occur without warning, regular checkups are important. Patients on long-term NSAIDs should have blood counts and liver enzymes checked periodically.

Unlike low-dose aspirin, there is little evidence that this or other NSAIDs will protect against heart attack or stroke. NSAIDs may be used with low-dose aspirin, but doing so may slightly increase your risk of gastric bleeding. Before taking this or any NSAID, tell your doctor if you take ACE inhibitors, lithium, warfarin or furosemide.

All NSAIDs may cause an increased risk of serious blood clots, heart attacks and stroke, which can be fatal. This risk may increase with dose and duration of use. Patients with cardiovascular disease or risk factors for cardiovascular disease may be at higher risk. These drugs should not be used for pain in people having coronary bypass surgery.

Allopurinol

Brand name(s):
Lopurin, Zyloprim

Type of Medication: Uric-acid-lowering drug

What it's used for: Gout

Dosage: 100 to 800 mg per day in a single dose. The dose is adjusted to have a serum uric acid level lower than 6 mg/dl.

Special instructions: Take immediately after a meal. Stop taking at the first sign of a rash, which may indicate an allergic reaction.

Possible side effects: Skin rash, hives or itching

Be aware: Before taking this drug, let your doctor know if you use azathioprine (*Imuran*) or if you have kidney disease. Acute gout attacks are common when this drug is started. These attacks can be minimized by taking lower doses and by taking the drug with colchicine or NSAIDs. Never start or stop allopurinol during a flare.

Amigesic

Generic name:
Salsalate

Other brand name(s):
Anaflex 750, Disalcid, Marthritic, Mono-Gesic, Salflex, Salsitab

Type of medication: NSAID, nonacetylated salicylate

What it's used for: to ease arthritis pain and inflammation

Dosage: 1,000 to 3,000 mg per day in 2 or 3 doses

Special instructions: Take with food. Do not chew tablets. Do not crush enteric-coated or time-release forms and mix with water. Do not combine with other NSAIDs.

Possible side effects: Abdominal or stomach cramps, pain or discomfort; diarrhea; dizziness; drowsiness or light-headedness; edema (swelling of the feet); headache; heartburn or indigestion; nausea or vomiting

Be aware: Dizziness, deafness or ringing in the ears indicates that you are taking too much. Before taking these medications, let your doctor know if you drink alcohol or use other NSAIDs. If you are taking doses of more than 3,600 mg per day, your doctor should monitor salicylate levels in your blood.

Amitriptyline hydrochloride

Brand name(s):
Endep

Type of medication: Antidepressant (tricyclic)

What it's used for: To relieve pain and promote sleep in fibromyalgia

Dosage: 10 to 80 mg per day in a single dose

Special instructions: Take at bedtime or several hours before bedtime to reduce "morning hangover."

Possible side effects: Constipation, dizziness, drowsiness, dry mouth, headache, tiredness, weight gain

Be aware: Before taking this medication, tell your doctor if you are using another antidepressant or have any of the following: a history of seizures, urinary retention, heart problems, or glaucoma or other chronic eye condition. Because adverse side effects can occur if you stop using this drug abruptly, discontinue it gradually. Know how you respond to this drug before driving or operating heavy machinery.

Anacin

Generic name:
Aspirin

Other brand name(s):
Ascriptin, Bayer, Bufferin, Ecotrin, Excedrin tablets

Type of medication: NSAID, salicylate (OTC)

What it's used for: To ease pain and inflammation associated with many forms of arthritis

Dosage: 2,400 to 5,400 mg per day in several doses

Special instructions: Take with food. Do not chew tablets; do not crush enteric-coated or time-release forms and mix with water. Do not combine with other NSAIDs.

Possible side effects: Abdominal or stomach cramps, pain or discomfort; diarrhea; dizziness, drowsiness or light-headedness; edema (swelling of the feet); headache; heartburn or indigestion; nausea or vomiting

Be aware: Ulcers and internal bleeding can occur without warning, so regular checkups are important. Confusion, deafness, dizziness or ringing in the ears indicates you are taking too much. Before taking this drug, let your doctor know if you drink alcohol, use blood thinners or have any of the following: sensitivity or allergy to aspirin or similar drugs, kidney disease, liver disease, asthma or peptic ulcers. If you are taking doses of more than 3,600 mg per day, your doctor should monitor the salicylate levels in your blood.

Anacin (aspirin-free)

Generic name:
acetaminophen

Other brand name(s):
Excedrin caplets, Panadol, Tylenol, Tylenol Arthritis Pain

Type of medication: Analgesic (OTC)

What it's used for: To relieve pain in any form of arthritis

Dosage: 325 to 1,000 mg every 4 to 6 hours as needed, no more than 4,000 mg per day

Special instructions: Do not use with any other product containing acetaminophen; do not use for more than 10 days for pain – unless directed by a doctor.

Possible side effects: When taken as directed, acetaminophen is usually not associated with side effects.

Be aware: If you consume 3 or more alcoholic drinks per day, consult your doctor before taking acetaminophen. Mixing acetaminophen with alcohol can cause liver damage.

Anaflex 750

Generic name:
Salsalate

Other brand name(s):
Amigesic, Disalcid, Marthritic, Mono-Gesic, Salflex, Salsitab

Type of medication: NSAID, nonacetylated salicylate

What it's used for: To ease arthritis pain and inflammation

Dosage: 1,000 to 3,000 mg per day in 2 or 3 doses

Special instructions: Take with food. Do not chew tablets. Do not crush enteric-coated or time-release forms and mix with water. Do not combine with other NSAIDs.

Possible side effects: Abdominal or stomach cramps, pain or discomfort; diarrhea; dizziness; drowsiness or light-headedness; edema (swelling of the feet); headache; heartburn or indigestion; nausea or vomiting

Be aware: Dizziness, deafness or ringing in the ears indicates that you are taking too much. Before taking these medications, let your doctor know if you drink alcohol or use other NSAIDs. If you are taking doses of more than 3,600 mg per day, your doctor should monitor salicylate levels in your blood.

Anakinra

Brand name(s):
Kineret

Type of medication: Biologic response modifier

What it's used for: To ease symptoms of rheumatoid arthritis and prevent joint damage

Dosage: 100 mg given once daily by subcutaneous (beneath the skin) injection; 100 mg every other day for patients with severe kidney disease

Special instructions: Refrigerate prior to use. Prefilled syringes can be self-injected with or without the aid of an automatic injector device (*SimpleJect*) available through the manufacturer. Do not shake. May be injected into the thigh, abdomen or upper arm. Try to administer at the same time every day.

Possible side effects: Injection site reactions (usually occurring during the first 4 to 6 weeks of use), including redness, swelling, pain and bruising; low white blood cell or platelet count; upper respiratory infection.

Be aware: Rheumatoid arthritis carries a higher risk of infection and lymphoma. It is uncertain whether this and other biologic response modifiers increase lymphoma risk. Discontinue if you have a serious infection (such as pneumonia) or recurrent infections. Do not take live vaccines; the flu vaccine or vaccine for pneumonia (*Pneumovax*) can be safely given.

Serious infections, such as pneumonia, occur in approximately 2 percent of people taking this drug. Inform your doctor if you have a current infection or history of serious infection.

Anaprox

Generic name:
Naproxen sodium

Other brand name(s):
Non-prescription: Aleve

Type of medication: NSAID

What it's used for: To ease arthritis pain and inflammation

Dosage: 550 to 1,650 mg per day in 2 doses

Special instructions: Do not take with other prescription or OTC NSAIDs. Take as directed at the same time(s) every day. If you experience stomach upset, take with food, a glass of milk or an antacid.

Possible side effects: Abdominal or stomach cramps, pain or discomfort; diarrhea; dizziness; drowsiness; edema (swelling of the feet); headache; gastrointestinal bleeding; heartburn or indigestion; nausea or vomiting; peptic ulcer.

Be aware: Before taking this medication, let your doctor know if you drink alcohol or use blood thinners or if you have or have had any of the following: sensitivity or allergy to aspirin or similar drugs, kidney or liver disease, heart disease, high blood pressure, asthma or stomach ulcers. Because stomach ulcers or internal bleeding can occur without warning, regular checkups are important.

Patients on long-term NSAIDs should have blood counts and liver enzymes checked periodically. Unlike low-dose aspirin, there is little evidence that this or other NSAIDs will protect against heart attack or stroke. NSAIDs may be used with low-dose aspirin, but doing so may slightly increase your risk of gastric bleeding. Before taking this or any NSAID, tell your doctor if you take ACE inhibitors, lithium, warfarin or furosemide.

All NSAIDs may cause an increased risk of serious blood clots, heart attacks and stroke, which can be fatal. This risk may increase with dose and duration of use. Patients with cardiovascular disease or risk factors for cardiovascular disease may be at higher risk. These drugs should not be used for pain in people having coronary bypass surgery.

Ansaid

Generic name:
Flurbiprofen

Type of medication: NSAID

What it's used for: To ease arthritis pain and inflammation

Dosage: 200 to 300 mg per day in 2 to 4 doses

Special instructions: Do not take with other prescription or OTC NSAIDs. Take as directed at the same time(s) every day. If you experience stomach upset, take with food, a glass of milk or an antacid.

Possible side effects: Abdominal or stomach cramps; pain or discomfort; diarrhea; dizziness; drowsiness; edema (swelling of the feet); gastrointestinal bleeding; headache; heartburn or indigestion; nausea or vomiting; peptic ulcer.

Be aware: Before taking this medication, let your doctor know if you drink alcohol or use blood thinners or if you have or have had any of the following: sensitivity or allergy to aspirin or similar drugs, kidney or liver disease, heart disease, high blood pressure, asthma or stomach ulcers. Because stomach ulcers or internal bleeding can occur without warning, regular checkups are important. Patients on long-term NSAIDs should have blood counts and liver enzymes checked periodically.

Unlike low-dose aspirin, there is little evidence that this or other NSAIDs will protect against heart attack or stroke. NSAIDs may be used with low-dose aspirin, but doing so may slightly increase your risk of gastric bleeding. Before taking this or any NSAID, tell your doctor if you take ACE inhibitors, lithium, warfarin or furosemide.

All NSAIDs may cause an increased risk of serious blood clots, heart attacks and stroke, which can be fatal. This risk may increase with dose and duration of use. Patients with cardiovascular disease or risk factors for cardiovascular disease may be at higher risk. These drugs should not be used for pain in people having coronary bypass surgery.

Arava

Generic name:
Leflunomide

Type of medication: DMARD

What it's used for: Rheumatoid arthritis

Dosage: 10 to 20 mg per day in a single dose

Special instructions: None.

Possible side effects: Dizziness, gastrointestinal problems, hair loss, headache, heartburn, high blood pressure, liver problems, low blood cell count, pain or burning in feet or hands (neuropathy), skin rash, stomach pain, sneezing, sore throat

Be aware: Do not use if pregnant. Before taking this medication, let your doctor know if you have active infection, liver or kidney disease or underlying cancer. Your doctor should order periodic tests to check for the drug's effect on the blood and liver. Either member of a couple who is taking leflunomide and is ready to conceive should go through an elimination process using the drug cholestyramine prior to conception.

Arthritab

Generic name:
Magnesium salicylate

Other brand name(s):
Prescription: Magan, Mobidin, Mobogesic
Non-prescription: Bayer Select, Doan's Pills

Type of medication: NSAID, nonacetylated salicylate (OTC)

What it's used for: To ease arthritis pain and inflammation

Dosage: 2,600 to 4,800 mg per day in 3 to 6 doses

Special instructions: Take with food. Do not chew tablets. Do not crush enteric-coated or time-release forms and mix with water. Do not combine with other NSAIDs.

Possible side effects: Abdominal or stomach cramps; pain or discomfort; diarrhea; dizziness; drowsiness or light-headedness; edema (swelling of the feet); headache; heartburn or indigestion; nausea or vomiting

Be aware: Dizziness, deafness or ringing in the ears indicates that you are taking too much. Before taking these medications, let your doctor know if you drink alcohol or use other NSAIDs. If you are taking doses of more than 3,600 mg per day, your doctor should monitor salicylate levels in your blood.

Arthropan

Generic name:
Choline salicylate (liquid only)

Type of medication: NSAID, nonacetylated-salicylate (OTC)

What it's used for: To ease arthritis pain and inflammation

Dosage: 3,480 mg or 20 mL per day in several doses

Special instructions: Do not combine with other NSAIDs.

Possible side effects: Abdominal or stomach cramps, pain or discomfort; diarrhea; dizziness; drowsiness or light-headedness; edema (swelling of the feet); headache; heartburn or indigestion; nausea or vomiting

Be aware: Dizziness, deafness or ringing in the ears indicates that you are taking too much. Before taking these medications, let your doctor know if you drink alcohol or use other NSAIDs. If you are taking doses of more than 3,600 mg per day, your doctor should monitor salicylate levels in your blood.

Arthrotec

Generic name:
Diclofenac sodium with misoprostol

Type of medication: NSAID plus prostaglandin substitute

What it's used for: To ease arthritis pain and inflammation; additional ingredient helps protect against NSAID-induced stomach ulcers

Dosage: 150 to 200 mg per day in 2 to 4 doses

Special instructions: Do not take with other prescription or OTC NSAIDs. Take as directed at the same times every day. If stomach upset occurs, take with food or a glass of milk.

Possible side effects: Abdominal or stomach cramps, pain or discomfort; diarrhea, dizziness; drowsiness; edema (swelling of feet); gastrointestinal bleeding; headache; heartburn or indigestion; nausea or vomiting; peptic ulcer. Note: Risk of gastric ulcers is less with this drug than with other NSAIDs. Risk of abdominal pain and diarrhea is greater with this drug.

Be aware: Before taking this medication, let your doctor know if you drink alcohol or use blood thinners, or if you have or have had any of the following: sensitivity or allergy to aspirin or similar drugs, kidney or liver disease, heart disease, high blood pressure, asthma or stomach ulcers. Because stomach ulcers or internal bleeding can occur without warning, regular checkups are important. Patients on long-term NSAIDs should have blood counts and liver enzymes checked periodically.

Unlike low-dose aspirin, there is little evidence that this or other NSAIDs will protect against heart attack or stroke. NSAIDs may be used with low-dose aspirin, but doing so may slightly increase your risk of gastric bleeding. Before taking this or any NSAID, tell your doctor if you take ACE inhibitors, lithium, warfarin or furosemide.

All NSAIDs may cause an increased risk of serious blood clots, heart attacks and stroke, which can be fatal. This risk may increase with dose and duration of use. Patients with cardiovascular disease or risk factors for cardiovascular disease may be at higher risk. These drugs should not be used for pain in people having coronary bypass surgery.

Ascriptin, see aspirin

Aspirin

Brand name(s):

Anacin, Ascriptin, Bayer, Bufferin, Ecotrin, Excedrin tablets

Type of medication: NSAIDs, salicylate (OTC)

What it's used for: To ease pain and inflammation associated with many forms of arthritis

Dosage: 2,400 to 5,400 mg per day in several doses

Special instructions: Take with food. Do not chew tablets; do not crush enteric-coated or time-release forms and mix with water. Do not combine with other NSAIDs.

Possible side effects: Abdominal or stomach cramps, pain or discomfort; diarrhea; dizziness, drowsiness or light-headedness; edema (swelling of the feet); headache; heartburn or indigestion; nausea or vomiting

Be aware: Ulcers and internal bleeding can occur without warning, so regular checkups are important. Confusion, deafness, dizziness or ringing in the ears indicates you are taking too much. Before taking this drug, let your doctor know if you drink alcohol, use blood thinners or have any of the following: sensitivity or allergy to aspirin or similar drugs, kidney disease, liver disease, asthma or peptic ulcers. If you are taking doses of more than 3,600 mg per day, your doctor should monitor the salicylate levels in your blood.

Auranofin (oral gold)

Brand name(s):
Ridaura

Type of medication: DMARD

What it's used for: Rheumatoid arthritis

Dosage: 6 to 9 mg per day in 1 or 2 doses

Special instructions: Take with a glass of milk or water. If stomach upset occurs, take with food.

Possible side effects: Diarrhea, low blood counts, metallic taste in mouth, mouth ulcers, protein in urine, skin rash or itching

Be aware: Before taking this drug, let your doctor know if you have or have had one of the following: adverse reaction to a gold-containing medication, a history of blood-cell abnormality, inflammatory bowel disease, or kidney or liver disease. This drug can cause sun sensitivity, so minimize exposure to sunlight and sunlamps and wear sunscreen. Your doctor should order periodic blood and urine tests to check for effects on the blood and kidneys.

Avinza

Generic name:
Morphine sulfate

Other brand name(s):
Oramorph SR

Type of medication: Analgesic

What it's used for: To ease severe pain associated with arthritis, surgery and fractures

Dosage: 30 mg per day in a single dose, to start; doctor may increase dose as necessary

Special instructions: Take at the same time each day with or without food. Swallow whole. Do not chew or crush. Do not stop drug abruptly. Do not drive or use heavy machinery until you know how your body reacts to this drug.

Possible side effects: Constipation, drowsiness, nausea

Be aware: Over time, this drug may cause psychological and physical dependence. Before taking this drug, let your doctor know if you use a central nervous system depressant, such antihistamines (allergy medications), tranquilizers, sleeping medications, muscle relaxants or narcotic pain medication, or if you have one of the following: liver disease, or history of alcohol or drug abuse.

Azathioprine

Brand name(s):
Imuran

Type of medication: DMARD

What it's used for: Rheumatoid arthritis, lupus and other autoimmune diseases

Dosage: 50 to 150 mg per day in 1 to 3 doses

Special instructions: Take with food.

Possible side effects: Fever or chills, loss of appetite, liver problems, low blood counts, nausea or vomiting, unusual tiredness or weakness

Be aware: Before taking this drug, tell your doctor if you use allopurinol or have kidney or liver disease. This drug can be associated with development of certain cancers, such as lymphoma. Your doctor may order periodic blood tests to check for effects on the blood.

Azulfidine

Generic name:
Sulfasalazine

Other brand name(s):
Azulfidine EN-Tabs

Type of medication: DMARD

What it's used for: Rheumatoid arthritis, lupus, ankylosing spondylitis and other forms of arthritis

Dosage: 500 to 3,000 mg per day in 2 to 4 doses

Possible side effects: Abdominal or stomach pain or upset, aching of joints, diarrhea, headache, increased sensitivity of skin to sunlight, itching, loss of appetite, nausea or vomiting, skin rash

Be aware: Let your doctor know if you have any of the following: allergy to sulfa drugs or aspirin, kidney or liver disease or blood disease. Failure to drink adequate fluids while on this medication can lead to the formation of urine crystals. This drug can lower sperm counts in men and may interfere with conception. Your doctor should order periodic blood tests to check for side effects of this drug.

Azulfidine EN-Tabs, see Azulfidine

Bayer

Generic name:
Aspirin

Other brand name(s):
Anacin, Ascriptin, Bufferin, Ecotrin, Excedrin tablets

Type of medication: NSAIDs, salicylate (OTC)

What it's used for: To ease pain and inflammation associated with many forms of arthritis

Dosage: 2,400 to 5,400 mg per day in several doses.

Special instructions: Take with food. Do not chew tablets; do not crush enteric-coated or time-release forms and mix with water. Do not combine with other NSAIDs.

Possible side effects: Abdominal or stomach cramps, pain or discomfort; diarrhea; dizziness, drowsiness or light-headedness; edema (swelling of the feet); headache; heartburn or indigestion; nausea or vomiting

Be aware: Ulcers and internal bleeding can occur without warning, so regular checkups are important. Confusion, deafness, dizziness or ringing in the ears indicates you are taking too much. Before taking this drug, let your doctor know if you drink alcohol, use blood thinners or have any of the following: sensitivity or allergy to aspirin or similar drugs, kidney disease, liver disease, asthma or peptic ulcers. If you are taking doses of more than 3,600 mg per day, your doctor should monitor the salicylate levels in your blood.

Bayer Select

Generic name:
Magnesium salicylate

Other brand name(s):
Prescription: Magan, Mobidin, Mobogesic
Non-prescription: Arthritab, Doan's Pills

Type of medication: NSAID, nonacetylated salicylate (OTC)

What it's used for: To ease arthritis pain and inflammation

Dosage: 2,600 to 4,800 mg per day in 3 to 6 doses

Special instructions: Take with food. Do not chew tablets. Do not crush enteric-coated or time-release forms and mix with water. Do not combine with other NSAIDs

Possible side effects: Abdominal or stomach cramps; pain or discomfort; diarrhea; dizziness; drowsiness or light-headedness; edema (swelling of the feet); headache; heartburn or indigestion; nausea or vomiting

Be aware: Dizziness, deafness or ringing in the ears indicates that you are taking too much. Before taking these medications, let your doctor know if you drink alcohol or use other NSAIDs. If you are taking doses of more than 3,600 mg per day, your doctor should monitor salicylate levels in your blood.

Benemid

Generic name:
Probenecid

Other brand name(s):
Probalan

Type of medication: Uric-acid-lowering medication

What it's used for: To reduce uric acid and decrease the frequency and severity of gout attacks

Dosage: 500 to 3,000 mg per day in 2 or 3 divided doses

Special instructions: Take with food or an antacid. Drink plenty of fluids. Do not take with aspirin or other NSAIDs. Avoid alcohol.

Possible side effects: Headache, loss of appetite, nausea or vomiting; stomach pain

Be aware: Before taking this drug, tell your doctor if you use cancer medications, heparin (calciparine, liguaemin), nitrofurantoin (*Furadantin, Macrobid, Macrodantin*), NSAIDs, or zidovudine (*Retrovir*), or if you have any of the following: blood disease, intestinal disease, kidney disease or kidney stones.

Betamethasone

Brand name (s):
Celestone, Celestone Soluspan

Type of medication: corticosteroid

What it's used for: to control inflammation of joints and organs in many forms of arthritis and related conditions

Dosage: Dosage varies widely according to the disease being treated. Taking either too much or too little can be dangerous. Take exactly the amount prescribed by your doctor.

Special instructions: Take with food. A single daily dose should be taken with breakfast. Sometimes the dose is split, taken 2 to 4 times per day. Don't stop medication abruptly; dosage must be tapered or reduced gradually.

Possible side effects: Bruising, cataracts, elevated blood sugars, hardening of the arteries (atherosclerosis), hypertension, increased appetite, indigestion, insomnia, mood swings, muscle weakness, nervousness or restlessness, osteoporosis, susceptibility to infection, thin skin

Be aware: Before taking this medication, let your doctor know if you have one of the following; fungal infection, history of tuberculosis, underactive thyroid, diabetes, stomach ulcer, high blood pressure or osteoporosis.

Boniva

Generic name:
ibandronate

Type of medication: Bisphosphonate

What it's used for: Postmenopausal osteoporosis

Dosage: 150 mg taken as a single monthly dose

Special instructions: Take only with one cup of water first thing in the morning. Swallow pill whole while sitting or standing; stay upright and avoid food for 60 minutes.

Possible side effects: Abdominal or stomach pain; heartburn

Be aware: Before taking this medication, tell your doctor if you are taking aspirin or aspirin-containing products, or if you have problems with the esophagus, stomach or kidneys. Blood levels of calcium and vitamin D must be normal before starting therapy.

Bufferin

Generic name:
Aspirin

Other brand name(s):
Anacin, Ascriptin, Bayer, Ecotrin, Excedrin tablets

Type of medication: NSAIDs, salicylate (OTC)

What it's used for: To ease pain and inflammation associated with many forms of arthritis

Dosage: 2,400 to 5,400 mg per day in several doses

Special instructions: Take with food. Do not chew tablets; do not crush enteric-coated or time-release forms and mix with water. Do not combine with other NSAIDs.

Possible side effects: Abdominal or stomach cramps, pain or discomfort; diarrhea; dizziness, drowsiness or light-headedness; edema (swelling of the feet); headache; heartburn or indigestion; nausea or vomiting

Be aware: Ulcers and internal bleeding can occur without warning, so regular checkups are important. Confusion, deafness, dizziness or ringing in the ears indicates you are taking too much. Before taking this drug, let your doctor know if you drink alcohol, use blood thinners or have any of the following: sensitivity or allergy to aspirin or similar drugs, kidney disease, liver disease, asthma or peptic ulcers. If you are taking doses of more than 3,600 mg per day, your doctor should monitor the salicylate levels in your blood.

Calcitonin

Brand name(s):
Miacalcin

Type of medication: Parathyroid hormone (nasal spray)

What it's used for: Osteoporosis

Dosage: 200 IUs per day in a single dose

Special instructions: Alternate nostrils daily. Store medication in refrigerator prior to opening. Store at room temperature after opening.

Possible side effects: Crusting, patches or sores inside the nose; dryness, itching, redness, swelling, tenderness or other signs of nasal irritation; nosebleeds; runny nose

Be aware: Before taking this drug, let your doctor know if you have a protein allergy.

Cataflam

Generic name:
Diclofenac potassium

Type of medication: NSAID

What it's used for: To ease arthritis pain and inflammation

Dosage: 100 to 200 mg per day in 2 or 4 doses

Special instructions: Do not take with other prescription or OTC NSAIDs. Take as directed at the same times every day. If stomach upset occurs, take with food, a glass of milk or an antacid.

Possible side effects: Abdominal or stomach cramps, pain or discomfort; diarrhea; dizziness; drowsiness; edema (swelling of feet); gastrointestinal bleeding; headache; heartburn or indigestion; nausea or vomiting; peptic ulcer

Be aware: Before taking this medication, let your doctor know if you drink alcohol or use blood thinners or if you have or have had any of the following: sensitivity or allergy to aspirin or similar drugs, kidney or liver disease, heart disease, high blood pressure, asthma or stomach ulcers. Because stomach ulcers or internal bleeding can occur without warning, regular checkups are important.

Unlike low-dose aspirin, there is little evidence that this or other NSAIDs will protect against heart attack or stroke. NSAIDs may be used with low-dose aspirin, but doing so may slightly increase your risk of gastric bleeding. Before taking this or any NSAID, tell your doctor if you take ACE inhibitors, lithium, warfarin or furosemide. Patients on long-term NSAIDs should have blood counts and liver enzymes checked periodically. Liver enzymes should be checked within four to eight weeks of starting the drug.

All NSAIDs may cause an increased risk of serious blood clots, heart attacks and stroke, which can be fatal. This risk may increase with dose and duration of use. Patients with cardiovascular disease or risk factors for cardiovascular disease may be at higher risk. These drugs should not be used for pain in people having coronary bypass surgery.

Celebrex

Generic name:
Celecoxib

Type of medication: NSAID (COX-2 inhibitor)

What it's used for: To ease arthritis pain and inflammation

Dosage: For ankylosing spondylitis or OA: 200 mg once per day or 100 mg twice per day; For RA: 100 to 200 mg twice per day

Special instructions: Do not take with other prescription or OTC NSAIDs.

Possible side effects: Abdominal or stomach cramps, pain or discomfort; diarrhea; dizziness, drowsiness; edema (swelling of the feet); gastrointestinal bleeding; headache; heartburn or indigestion; nausea or vomiting; peptic ulcer. Less likely to cause bleeding stomach ulcers and susceptibility to bruising or bleeding than traditional NSAIDs.

Be aware: Unlike low-dose aspirin, there is no evidence this drug will protect against heart attack or stroke. This drug may be used with low-dose aspirin, but may slightly increase your ulcer risk. Before taking this drug, tell your doctor if you have had a heart attack, stroke, angina, blood clot, hypertension or sensitivity to aspirin or other NSAIDs. Also, tell your doctor if you have sensitivity to sulfonamides, a type of sulfa drug, or to aspirin or other arthritis medications.

All NSAIDs may cause an increased risk of serious blood clots, heart attacks and stroke, which can be fatal. This risk may increase with dose and duration of use. Patients with cardiovascular disease or risk factors for cardiovascular disease may be at higher risk. These drugs should not be used for pain in people having coronary bypass surgery.

Celecoxib

Brand name(s):
Celebrex

Type of medication: NSAID (COX-2 inhibitor)

What it's used for: To ease arthritis pain and inflammation

Dosage: For ankylosing spondylitis or OA: 200 mg once per day or 100 mg twice per day; For RA: 100 to 200 mg twice per week

Special instructions: Do not take with other prescription or OTC NSAIDs.

Possible side effects: Abdominal or stomach cramps, pain or discomfort; diarrhea; dizziness, drowsiness; edema (swelling of the feet); gastrointestinal bleeding; headache; heartburn or indigestion; nausea or vomiting; peptic ulcer. Less likely to cause bleeding stomach ulcers and susceptibility to bruising or bleeding than traditional NSAIDs.

Be aware: Unlike low-dose aspirin, there is no evidence this drug will protect against heart attack or stroke. This drug may be used with low-dose aspirin, but may slightly increase your ulcer risk. Before taking this drug, tell your doctor if you have had a heart attack, stroke, angina, blood clot, hypertension, or sensitivity to aspirin or other NSAIDs. Also, tell your doctor if you have sensitivity to sulfonamides, a type of sulfa drug, or to aspirin or other arthritis medications.

All NSAIDs may cause an increased risk of serious blood clots, heart attacks and stroke, which can be fatal. This risk may increase with dose and duration of use. Patients with cardiovascular disease or risk factors for cardiovascular disease may be at higher risk. These drugs should not be used for pain in people having coronary bypass surgery.

Celestone

Generic name:
betamethasone

Other brand name(s):
Celestone Soluspan

Type of medication: corticosteroid

What it's used for: to control inflammation of joints and organs in many forms of arthritis and related conditions

Dosage: Dosage varies widely according to the disease being treated. Taking either too much or too little can be dangerous. Take exactly the amount prescribed by your doctor.

Special instructions: Take with food. A single daily dose should be taken with breakfast. Sometimes the dose is split, taken 2 to 4 times per day. Don't stop medication abruptly; dosage must be tapered or reduced gradually.

Possible side effects: Bruising, cataracts, elevated blood sugars, hardening of the arteries (atherosclerosis), hypertension, increased appetite, indigestion, insomnia, mood swings, muscle weakness, nervousness or restlessness, osteoporosis, susceptibility to infection, thin skin.

Be aware: Before taking this medication, let your doctor know if you have one of the following; fungal infection, history of tuberculosis, underactive thyroid, diabetes, stomach ulcer, high blood pressure or osteoporosis.

Celestone Soluspan, See betamethasone

Chlorambucil

Brand name(s):
Leukeran

Type of medication: DMARD

What it's used for: Severe rheumatoid arthritis; lupus kidney disease

Dosage: 2 to 8 mg per day in 1 or 2 doses

Special instructions: Use only for life-threatening organ disease.

Possible side effects: Hair loss, low blood counts, missing menstrual periods, nausea

Be aware: Let your doctor know if you have active infection. Use of this drug may make you more susceptible to infections and certain cancers.

Choline and magnesium salicylates

Brand name(s):
CMT, Tricosal, Trilisate

Type of medication: NSAID (nonacetylated salicylate)

What it's used for: To ease arthritis pain and inflammation

Dosage: 2,000 to 3,000 mg per day in 2 or 3 doses

Special instructions: Take with food. Do not chew tablets. Do not crush enteric-coated or time-release forms and mix with water. Do not combine with other NSAIDs.

Possible side effects: Abdominal or stomach cramps, pain or discomfort; diarrhea; dizziness, drowsiness or light-headedness; edema (swelling of the feet); headache; heartburn or indigestion; nausea or vomiting

Be aware: Dizziness, deafness or ringing in the ears indicates that you are taking too much. Before taking this medication, let your doctor know if you drink alcohol or use other NSAIDs. If you are taking doses of more than 3,600 mg per day, your doctor should monitor salicylate levels in your blood.

Choline salicylate (liquid only)

Brand name(s):
Arthropan

Type of medication: NSAID (nonacetylated-salicylate)

What it's used for: To ease arthritis pain and inflammation

Dosage: 3,480 mg or 20 mL per day in several doses

Special instructions: Do not combine with other NSAIDs.

Possible side effects: Abdominal or stomach cramps, pain or discomfort; diarrhea; dizziness, drowsiness or light-headedness; edema (swelling of the feet); headache; heartburn or indigestion; nausea or vomiting

Be aware: Dizziness, deafness or ringing in the ears indicates that you are taking too much. Before taking these medications, let your doctor know if you drink alcohol or use other NSAIDs. If you are taking doses of more than 3,600 mg per day, your doctor should monitor salicylate levels in your blood.

Clinoril

Generic name:
Sulindac

Type of medication: NSAID

What it's used for: To ease arthritis pain and inflammation

Dosage: 300 to 400 mg per day in 2 doses

Special instructions: Do not take with other prescription or OTC NSAIDs. Take as directed at the same time(s) every day. If you experience stomach upset, take with food, a glass of milk or an antacid.

Possible side effects: Abdominal or stomach cramps, pain or discomfort; diarrhea; dizziness; edema (swelling of the feet); headache; gastrointestinal bleeding; heartburn or indigestion; nausea or vomiting; peptic ulcer

Be aware: Before taking this medication, let your doctor know if you drink alcohol or use blood thinners, or if you have or have had any of the following: sensitivity or allergy to aspirin or similar drugs, kidney or liver disease, heart disease, high blood pressure, asthma or stomach ulcers. Because stomach ulcers or internal bleeding can occur without warning, regular checkups are important. Patients on long-term NSAIDs should have blood counts and liver enzymes checked periodically.

Unlike low-dose aspirin, there is little evidence that this or other NSAIDs will protect against heart attack or stroke. NSAIDs may be used with low-dose aspirin, but doing so may slightly increase your risk of gastric bleeding. Before taking this or any NSAID, tell your doctor if you take ACE inhibitors, lithium, warfarin or furosemide.

All NSAIDs may cause an increased risk of serious blood clots, heart attacks and stroke, which can be fatal. This risk may increase with dose and duration of use. Patients with cardiovascular disease or risk factors for cardiovascular disease may be at higher risk. These drugs should not be used for pain in people having coronary bypass surgery.

Civemeline

Brand name(s):
Evoxac

Type of medication: Cholinergic agonist

What it's used for: To increase saliva production, relieve dry mouth associated with Sjögren's syndrome

Dosage: 30 mg 3 times per day

Special instructions: Start with a low dose and take after meals to minimize side effects. Allow 6 to 12 weeks of uninterrupted treatment before improvement.

Possible side effects: Changes in heart rate (rare); diarrhea; excessive sweating; problems with night vision; nausea; rhinitis

Be aware: Do not take if you have uncontrolled asthma, chronic bronchitis, chronic obstructive pulmonary disease, significant cardiovascular disease, acute iritis or narrow-angle glaucoma. Let your doctor know if you take beta adrenergic antagonists (betablockers).

CMT

Generic name:
Choline and magnesium salicylates
Other brand name(s):
Tricosal, Trilisate

Type of medication: NSAID (nonacetylated salicylate)

What it's used for: To ease arthritis pain and inflammation

Dosage: 2,000 to 3,000 mg per day in 2 or 3 doses

Special instructions: Take with food. Do not chew tablets. Do not crush enteric-coated or time-release forms and mix with water. Do not combine with other NSAIDs.

Possible side effects: Abdominal or stomach cramps, pain or discomfort; diarrhea; dizziness, drowsiness or light-headedness; edema (swelling of the feet); headache; heartburn or indigestion; nausea or vomiting

Be aware: Dizziness, deafness or ringing in the ears indicates that you are taking too much. Before taking this medication, let your doctor know if you drink alcohol or use other NSAIDs. If you are taking doses of more than 3,600 mg per day, your doctor should monitor salicylate levels in your blood.

ColBenemid, see probenecid and colchicine

Colchicine

Brand name(s):
Available only as a generic

Type of medication: Anti-inflammatory

What it's used for: To prevent or ease gout attacks

Dosage: 0.6 to 1.2 mg per day in 1 or 2 doses for prevention; 0.6 mg every 1 or 2 hours (no more than 8 doses per day) to stop acute attacks

Special instructions: Take with food if stomach upset occurs. Drink plenty of fluids.

Possible side effects: Diarrhea, nausea or vomiting, pain or burning in feet or hands (neuropathy), stomach pain

Be aware: Before taking this drug, tell your doctor if you have intestinal, kidney or liver disease. Special caution is required in people who have an ongoing infection or are using immunosuppressive drugs.

Col-Probenecid, see Probenecid and colchicine

Cortef

Generic name:
Hydrocortisone

Other brand name(s):
Hydrocortone

Type of medication: Corticosteroid

What it's used for: To control inflammation of joints and organs in many forms of arthritis and related conditions

Dosage: Dosage varies widely according to the disease being treated. Taking either too much or too little can be dangerous. Take exactly the amount prescribed by your doctor.

Special instructions: Take with food. A single daily dose should be taken with breakfast. Sometimes the dose is split, taken 2 to 4 times per day. Don't stop medication abruptly; dosage must be tapered or reduced gradually.

Possible side effects: Bruising, cataracts, elevated blood fats (cholesterol, triglycerides), elevated blood sugar, hardening of the arteries (atherosclerosis), hypertension, increased appetite, indigestion, insomnia, mood swings, muscle weakness, nervousness or restlessness, osteoporosis, susceptibility to infection, thin skin

Be aware: Before taking this medication, let your doctor know if you have one of the following: fungal infection, history of tuberculosis, underactive thyroid, diabetes, stomach ulcer, high blood pressure or osteoporosis.

Cortisone acetate

Brand name(s):
Cortone

Type of medication: Corticosteroid

What it's used for: To control inflammation of joints and organs in many forms of arthritis and related conditions

Dosage: Dosage varies widely according to the disease being treated. Taking either too much or too little can be dangerous. Take exactly the amount prescribed by your doctor.

Special instructions: Take with food. A single daily dose should be taken with breakfast. Sometimes the dose is split, taken 2 to 4 times per day. Don't stop medication abruptly; dosage must be tapered or reduced gradually.

Possible side effects: Bruising, cataracts, elevated blood fats (cholesterol, triglycerides), elevated blood sugar, hardening of the arteries (atherosclerosis), hypertension, increased appetite, indigestion, insomnia, mood swings, muscle weakness, nervousness or restlessness, osteoporosis, susceptibility to infection, thin skin

Be aware: Before taking this medication, let your doctor know if you have one of the following: fungal infection, history of tuberculosis, underactive thyroid, diabetes, stomach ulcer, high blood pressure or osteoporosis.

Cortone, see **Cortisone acetate**

Cuprimine

Generic name:
Penicillamine

Brand name(s):
Depen

Type of medication: DMARD

What it's used for: Rheumatoid arthritis

Dosage: 125 to 250 mg per day in a single dose to start, increased to not more than 1,500 mg per day in 3 doses

Special instructions: Take on an empty stomach, at least 1 hour before or 2 hours after any food, milk or medicine.

Possible side effects: Abdominal pain or upset, diarrhea, flushing, headache, increased sun sensitivity, itching, joint pain, loss of appetite, nausea or vomiting, skin rash

Be aware: Before taking this medication, let your doctor know if you have any of the following: penicillin allergy, blood disease, kidney disease or lupus. Because this drug can cause blood abnormalities and kidney damage, your doctor should order periodic blood and urine tests to check for unwanted effects. Take consistently; stopping and starting can worsen side effects.

Cyclobenzaprine

Brand name(s):
Cycloflex, Flexeril

Type of medication: Muscle relaxant

What it's used for: To promote sleep and ease muscle pain in fibromyalgia

Dosage: 5 to 30 mg per day in a single dose

Special instructions: Take 2 to 3 hours before bedtime to reduce "morning hangover."

Possible side effects: blurred vision, dizziness or light-headedness, drowsiness, dry mouth

Be aware: Before taking this medication, let your doctor know if you use alcohol or other central nervous system (CNS) depressants such as antihistamines, cold or allergy medications, tranquilizers, sleeping medications, muscle relaxants or narcotic pain medication, or if you have any of the following: glaucoma, problems with urination, heart or blood vessel disease or overactive thyroid.

Cycloflex, see Cyclobenzaprine

Cyclophosphamide

Brand name(s):
Cytoxan

Type of medication: DMARD

What it's used for: Severe rheumatoid arthritis or lupus affecting internal organs

Dosage: 50 to 150 mg per day in a single dose orally (this drug may also be given intravenously)

Special instructions: Take oral medication with breakfast. Drink lots of fluids throughout the day and empty bladder before bedtime. Use only for severe organ disease.

Possible side effects: Blood in urine; darkening of skin and fingernails; hair loss; infertility; loss of appetite; low blood counts; missing menstrual periods; nausea or vomiting

Be aware: Tell your doctor if you have liver or kidney disease, an active infection or high blood pressure. Use of this drug may make you more susceptible to infection and certain cancers. Your doctor should order periodic tests to check for side effects of this drug on the blood and urinary tract.

Cyclosporine

Brand name(s):
Neoral

Type of medication: DMARD

What it's used for: To slow the progression of rheumatoid arthritis

Dosage: 100 to 400 mg per day in 2 doses. Exact doses vary by weight.

Special instructions: Take at the same times every day, either with meals or between meals.

Possible side effects: Headache, high blood pressure, increase in hair growth, kidney problems, loss of appetite, nausea

Be aware: Before taking this drug, tell your doctor if you have liver or kidney disease, active infection or high blood pressure. Because this drug's rate of absorption is unpredictable, your doctor should monitor it through blood tests. Use of this drug may make you more susceptible to infection and certain cancers. Do not take with St. John's wort, grapefruit or grapefruit juice.

Cyclosporine ophthalmic emulsion

Brand name(s):
Restasis

Type of medication: Immunosuppressive/eye drop

What it's used for: To relieve dry eyes associated with Sjögren's syndrome

Dosage: One drop in each eye twice per day, approximately 12 hours apart

Special instructions: Single-use vials must be used immediately upon opening and then discarded.

Possible side effects: Blurred vision; burning, pain, itching or stinging feelings in eye; discharge; foreign body sensation

Be aware: Cyclosporine is an immunosuppressant. Do not use if you have an eye infection. Do not wear contact lenses while using this medication.

Cymbalta

Generic name:
Duloxetine

Type of medication: Antidepressant [selective serotonin and norepinephrine reuptake inhibitor (SSNRI)]

What it's used for: To improve depression, relieve fatigue and improve energy in people with fibromyalgia

Dosage: 60 mg twice daily

Special instructions: Build dose gradually; taper dose slowly

Possible side effects: Anxiety or nervousness; constipation; decrease in sexual desire or ability; decreased appetite; diarrhea; drowsiness; dry mouth; headache; hives or itching; increased sweating; nausea; restlessness; skin rash; tiredness or weakness; trembling or shaking; trouble sleeping. Side effects may continue after treatment is stopped.

Be aware: Combining this drug with alcohol or other central nervous system depressants (including antihistamines, narcotic medications and some dental anesthetics) can increase their effects and side effects. Taking with aspirin or other NSAIDs may increase risk of bleeding. Never stop taking this medication abruptly. Your doctor will taper your dosage gradually. Do not take within 14 days of taking a monoamine oxidase (MAO) inhibitor. Patients and their family members should be aware of agitation and suicidal tendencies.

Cytoxan

Generic name:
Cyclophosphamide

Type of medication: DMARD

What it's used for: Severe rheumatoid arthritis or lupus affecting internal organs

Dosage: 50 to 150 mg per day in a single dose orally (this drug may also be given intravenously)

Special instructions: Take oral medication with breakfast. Drink lots of fluids throughout the day and empty bladder before bedtime. Use only for severe organ disease.

Possible side effects: Blood in urine; darkening of skin and fingernails; hair loss; infertility; loss of appetite; low blood counts; missing menstrual periods; nausea or vomiting

Be aware: Tell your doctor if you have liver or kidney disease, an active infection or high blood pressure. Use of this drug may make you more susceptible to infection and certain cancers. Your doctor should order periodic tests to check for side effects of this drug on the blood and urinary tract.

Darvocet

Generic name:
Propoxyphene with acetaminophen

Type of medication: Analgesic

What it's used for: Severe pain from arthritis, surgery or fractures

Dosage: 50 to 100 mg propoxyphene (325 to 650 mg acetaminophen) every 4 hours as needed, not to exceed 600 mg propoxyphene per day

Special instructions: Never take more of this drug than your doctor prescribes. Do not increase dose on your own because side effects increase and tolerance develops as dosage increases; do not drive or operate heavy machinery until you know how your body reacts to this drug.

Possible side effects: Dizziness, nausea, sedation, vomiting

Be aware: If you consume 3 or more alcoholic drinks per day, consult your doctor before taking this medication. Acetaminophen can cause liver damage. Mixing acetaminophen with alcohol can cause liver damage.

Over time, this drug may cause psychological and physical dependence. Before taking this drug, let your doctor know if you use a central nervous system depressant, such as antihistamines (allergy medications), tranquilizers, sleeping medications, muscle relaxants or narcotic pain medications, or if you have one of the following: liver disease, or history of alcohol or drug abuse. Avoid taking more than one product containing acetaminophen.

Darvon

Generic name:
Propoxyphene hydrochloride

Other brand name(s):
PP-Cap

Type of medication: Analgesic

What it's used for: Severe pain from arthritis, surgery or fractures

Dosage: 65 mg every 4 hours as needed, no more than 390 mg per day

Special instructions: Never take more of this drug than your doctor prescribes. Do not increase dose on your own because side effects increase and tolerance develops as dosage increases; do not drive or operate heavy machinery until you know how your body reacts to this drug.

Possible side effects: Dizziness, nausea, sedation, vomiting

Be aware: Over time, this drug may cause psychological and physical dependence. Before taking this drug, let your doctor know if you use a central nervous system depressant, such as antihistamines (allergy medications), tranquilizers, sleeping medications, muscle relaxants or narcotic pain medications, or if you have one of the following: liver disease, or history of alcohol or drug abuse.

Daypro

Generic name:
Oxaprozin

Type of medication: NSAID

What it's used for: To ease arthritis pain and inflammation

Dosage: 1,200 or 1,800 mg per day in a single dose

Special instructions: Do not take with other prescription or OTC NSAIDs. Take as directed at the same time every day. If you experience stomach upset, take with food or a glass of milk.

Possible side effects: Abdominal or stomach cramps, pain or discomfort; diarrhea; dizziness; edema (swelling of the feet); gastrointestinal bleeding; headache; heartburn or indigestion; nausea or vomiting; peptic ulcer

Be aware: Before taking this medication, let your doctor know if you drink alcohol or use blood thinners or if you have or have had any of the following: sensitivity or allergy to aspirin or similar drugs, kidney or liver disease, heart disease, high blood pressure, asthma or stomach ulcers. Because stomach ulcers or internal bleeding can occur without warning, regular checkups are important. Patients on long-term NSAIDs should have blood counts and liver enzymes checked periodically.

Unlike low-dose aspirin, there is little evidence that this or other NSAIDs will protect against heart attack or stroke. NSAIDs may be used with low-dose aspirin, but doing so may slightly increase your risk of gastric bleeding. Before taking this or any NSAID, tell your doctor if you take ACE inhibitors, lithium, warfarin or furosemide.

All NSAIDs may cause an increased risk of serious blood clots, heart attacks and stroke, which can be fatal. This risk may increase with dose and duration of use. Patients with cardiovascular disease or risk factors for cardiovascular disease may be at higher risk. These drugs should not be used for pain in people having coronary bypass surgery.

Decadron

Generic name:
Dexamethasone

Other brand name(s):
Hexadrol

Type of medication: Corticosteroid

What it's used for: To control inflammation of joints and organs in many forms of arthritis and related conditions

Dosage: Dosage varies widely according to the disease being treated. Taking either too much or too little can be dangerous. Take exactly the amount prescribed by your doctor.

Special instructions: Take with food. A single daily dose should be taken with breakfast. Sometimes the dose is split, taken 2 to 4 times per day. Don't stop medication abruptly; dosage must be tapered or reduced gradually.

Possible side effects: Bruising, cataracts, elevated blood fats (cholesterol, triglycerides), elevated blood sugar, hardening of the arteries (atherosclerosis), hypertension, increased appetite, indigestion, insomnia, mood swings, muscle weakness, nervousness or restlessness, osteoporosis, susceptibility to infection, thin skin

Be aware: Before taking this medication, let your doctor know if you have one of the following: fungal infection, history of tuberculosis, underactive thyroid, diabetes, stomach ulcer, high blood pressure or osteoporosis.

Deltasone

Generic name:
Prednisone

Other brand name(s):
Orasone, Prednicen-M, Sterapred

Type of medication: Corticosteroid

What it's used for: To control inflammation of joints and organs in many forms of arthritis and related conditions

Dosage: Dosage varies widely according to the disease being treated. Taking either too much or too little can be dangerous. Take exactly the amount prescribed by your doctor.

Special instructions: Take with food. A single daily dose should be taken with breakfast. Sometimes the dose is split, taken 2 to 4 times per day. Don't stop medication abruptly; dosage must be tapered or reduced gradually.

Possible side effects: Bruising, cataracts, elevated blood fats (cholesterol, triglycerides), elevated blood sugar, hardening of the arteries (atherosclerosis), hypertension, increased appetite, indigestion, insomnia, mood swings, muscle weakness, nervousness or restlessness, osteoporosis, susceptibility to infection, thin skin

Be aware: Before taking this medication, let your doctor know if you have one of the following: fungal infection, history of tuberculosis, underactive thyroid, diabetes, stomach ulcer, high blood pressure or osteoporosis.

Depen

Generic name:
Penicillamine

Other brand name(s):
Cuprimine

Type of medication: DMARD

What it's used for: Rheumatoid arthritis

Dosage: 125 to 250 mg per day in a single dose to start, increased to not more than 1,500 mg per day in 3 doses

Special instructions: Take on an empty stomach at least 1 hour before or 2 hours after any food, milk or medicine.

Possible side effects: Abdominal pain or upset; aching of joints; diarrhea; flushing; headache; increased sun sensitivity; itching; joint pain; loss of appetite; nausea or vomiting; skin rash

Be aware: Before taking this medication, let your doctor know if you have any of the following: penicillin allergy, blood disease, kidney disease or lupus. Because this drug can cause blood abnormalities and kidney damage, your doctor should order periodic blood and urine tests to check for unwanted effects. Take consistently; stopping and starting can worsen side effects.

Dexamethasone

Brand name(s):
Decadron, Hexadrol

Type of medication: Corticosteroid

What it's used for: To control inflammation of joints and organs in many forms of arthritis and related conditions

Dosage: Dosage varies widely according to the disease being treated. Taking either too much or too little can be dangerous. Take exactly the amount prescribed by your doctor.

Special instructions: Take with food. A single daily dose should be taken with breakfast. Sometimes the dose is split, taken 2 to 4 times per day. Don't stop medication abruptly; dosage must be tapered or reduced gradually.

Possible side effects: Bruising, cataracts, elevated blood fats (cholesterol, triglycerides), elevated blood sugar, hardening of the arteries (atherosclerosis), hypertension, increased appetite, indigestion, insomnia, mood swings, muscle weakness, nervousness or restlessness, osteoporosis, susceptibility to infection, thin skin

Be aware: Before taking this medication, let your doctor know if you have one of the following: fungal infection, history of tuberculosis, underactive thyroid, diabetes, stomach ulcer, high blood pressure or osteoporosis.

Diclofenac potassium

Brand name(s):
Cataflam

Type of medication: NSAID

What it's used for: To ease arthritis pain and inflammation

Dosage: 100 to 200 mg per day in 2 or 4 doses

Special instructions: Do not take with other prescription or OTC NSAIDs. Take as directed at the same times every day. If stomach upset occurs, take with food, a glass of milk or an antacid.

Possible side effects: Abdominal or stomach cramps, pain or discomfort; diarrhea; dizziness; edema (swelling of feet); gastrointestinal bleeding; headache; heartburn or indigestion; nausea or vomiting; peptic ulcer

Be aware: Before taking this medication, let your doctor know if you drink alcohol or use blood thinners or if you have or have had any of the following: sensitivity or allergy to aspirin or similar drugs, kidney or liver disease, heart disease, high blood pressure, asthma or stomach ulcers. Because stomach ulcers or internal bleeding can occur without warning, regular checkups are important. Patients on long-term NSAIDs should have blood counts and liver enzymes checked periodically. Liver enzymes should be checked within 4 to 8 weeks of starting the drug.

Unlike low-dose aspirin, there is little evidence that this or other NSAIDs will protect against heart attack or stroke. NSAIDs may be used with low-dose aspirin, but doing so may slightly increase your risk of gastric bleeding. Before taking this or any NSAID, tell your doctor if you take ACE inhibitors, lithium, warfarin or furosemide.

All NSAIDs may cause an increased risk of serious blood clots, heart attacks and stroke, which can be fatal. This risk may increase with dose and duration of use. Patients with cardiovascular disease or risk factors for cardiovascular disease may be at higher risk. These drugs should not be used for pain in people having coronary bypass surgery.

Diclofenac sodium

Brand name(s):
Voltaren, Voltaren-XR

Type of medication: NSAID

What it's used for: To control arthritis pain and inflammation

Dosage: 100 to 200 mg per day in 2 or 4 doses (*Voltaren*); 100 mg per day in a single dose (*Voltaren-XR*)

Special instructions: Do not take with other prescription or OTC NSAIDs. Take as directed at the same time every day. If stomach upset occurs, take with food, a glass of milk or an antacid.

Possible side effects: Abdominal or stomach cramps, pain or discomfort; diarrhea; dizziness; drowsiness; edema (swelling of feet); gastrointestinal bleeding; headache; heartburn or indigestion; nausea or vomiting; peptic ulcer

Be aware: Before taking this medication, let your doctor know if you drink alcohol or use blood thinners, or if you have or have had any of the following: sensitivity or allergy to aspirin or similar drugs, kidney or liver disease, heart disease, high blood pressure, asthma or stomach ulcers. Because stomach ulcers or internal bleeding can occur without warning, regular checkups are important. Patients on long-term NSAIDs should have blood counts and liver enzymes checked periodically. Liver enzymes should be checked within 4 to 8 weeks of starting the drug.

Unlike low-dose aspirin, there is little evidence that this or other NSAIDs will protect against heart attack or stroke. NSAIDs may be used with low-dose aspirin, but doing so may slightly increase your risk of gastric bleeding. Before taking this or any NSAID, tell your doctor if you take ACE inhibitors, lithium, warfarin or furosemide.

All NSAIDs may cause an increased risk of serious blood clots, heart attacks and stroke, which can be fatal. This risk may increase with dose and duration of use. Patients with cardiovascular disease or risk factors for cardiovascular disease may be at higher risk. These drugs should not be used for pain in people having coronary bypass surgery.

Diclofenac sodium with misoprostol

Brand name(s):
Arthrotec

Type of medication: NSAID (plus prostaglandin substitute)

What it's used for: To ease arthritis pain and inflammation; additional ingredient helps protect against NSAID-induced stomach ulcers

Dosage: 150 to 200 mg per day in 2 to 4 doses

Special instructions: Do not take with other prescription or OTC NSAIDs. Take as directed at the same times every day. If stomach upset occurs, take with food, a glass of milk or an antacid.

Possible side effects: Abdominal or stomach cramps, pain or discomfort; diarrhea; dizziness; light-headedness; edema (swelling of feet); gastrointestinal bleeding: headache; heartburn or indigestion; nausea or vomiting; peptic ulcer. Note: risk of gastric ulcers is less with this drug than with other NSAIDs. Risk of abdominal pain and diarrhea is greater with this drug.

Be aware: Before taking this medication, let your doctor know if you drink alcohol or use blood thinners, or if you have or have had any of the following: sensitivity or allergy to aspirin or similar drugs, kidney or liver disease, heart disease, high blood pressure, asthma or stomach ulcers. Because stomach ulcers or internal bleeding can occur

without warning, regular checkups are important. Patients on long-term NSAIDs should have blood counts and liver enzymes checked periodically.

Unlike low-dose aspirin, there is little evidence that this or other NSAIDs will protect against heart attack or stroke. NSAIDs may be used with low-dose aspirin, but doing so may slightly increase your risk of gastric bleeding. Before taking this or any NSAID, tell your doctor if you take ACE inhibitors, lithium, warfarin or furosemide.

All NSAIDs may cause an increased risk of serious blood clots, heart attacks and stroke, which can be fatal. This risk may increase with dose and duration of use. Patients with cardiovascular disease or risk factors for cardiovascular disease may be at higher risk. These drugs should not be used for pain in people having coronary bypass surgery.

Diflunisal

Brand name(s):
Dolobid

Type of medication: NSAID

What it's used for: To ease arthritis pain and inflammation

Dosage: 500 to 1,500 mg per day in 2 doses

Special instructions: Do not take with other prescription or OTC NSAIDs. Take as directed at the same times every day. If you experience stomach upset, take with food, a glass of milk or an antacid.

Possible side effects: Abdominal or stomach cramps, pain or discomfort; diarrhea; dizziness; light-headedness; edema (swelling of feet); gastrointestinal bleeding: headache; heartburn or indigestion; nausea or vomiting; peptic ulcer

Be aware: Before taking this medication, let your doctor know if you drink alcohol or use blood thinners, or if you have or have had any of the following: sensitivity or allergy to aspirin or similar drugs, kidney or liver disease, heart disease, high blood pressure, asthma or stomach ulcers. Because stomach ulcers or internal bleeding can occur without warning, regular checkups are important. Patients on long-term NSAIDs should have blood counts and liver enzymes checked periodically.

Unlike low-dose aspirin, there is little evidence that this or other NSAIDs will protect against heart attack or stroke. NSAIDs may be used with low-dose aspirin, but doing so may slightly increase your risk of gastric bleeding. Before taking this or any NSAID, tell your doctor if you take ACE inhibitors, lithium, warfarin or furosemide.

All NSAIDs may cause an increased risk of serious blood clots, heart attacks and stroke, which can be fatal. This risk may increase with dose and duration of use. Patients with cardiovascular disease or risk factors for cardiovascular disease may be at higher risk. These drugs should not be used for pain in people having coronary bypass surgery.

Disalcid

Generic name:
Salsalate

Other brand name(s):
Amigesic, Anaflex 750, Marthritic, Mono-Gesic, Salflex, Salsitab

Type of medication: NSAID (nonacetylated salicylate)

What it's used for: To ease arthritis pain and inflammation

Dosage: 1,000 to 3,000 mg per day in 2 or 3 doses

Special instructions: Take with food. Do not chew tablets. Do not crush enteric-coated or time-release forms and mix with water. Do not combine with other NSAIDs.

Possible side effects: Abdominal or stomach cramps, pain or discomfort; diarrhea; dizziness; drowsiness or light-headedness; edema (swelling of the feet); headache; heartburn or indigestion; nausea or vomiting

Be aware: Dizziness, deafness or ringing in the ears indicates that you are taking too much. Before taking these medications, let your doctor know if you drink alcohol or use other NSAIDs. If you are taking doses of more than 3,600 mg per day, your doctor should monitor salicylate levels in your blood.

Doan's Pills

Generic name:
Magnesium salicylate

Other brand name(s):
Prescription: Magan, Mobidin, Mobogesic
Non-prescription: Arthritab, Bayer Select

Type of medication: NSAID, nonacetylated salicylate (OTC)

What it's used for: To ease arthritis pain and inflammation

Dosage: 2,600 to 4,800 mg per day in 3 to 6 doses

Special instructions: Take with food. Do not chew tablets. Do not crush enteric-coated or time-release forms and mix with water. Do not combine with other NSAIDs.

Possible side effects: Abdominal or stomach cramps, pain or discomfort; diarrhea; dizziness; drowsiness or light-headedness; edema (swelling of the feet); headache; heartburn or indigestion; nausea or vomiting

Be aware: Dizziness, deafness or ringing in the ears indicates that you are taking too much. Before taking these medications, let your doctor know if you drink alcohol or use other NSAIDs. If you are taking doses of more than 3,600 mg per day, your doctor should monitor salicylate levels in your blood.

Dolobid

Generic name:
Diflunisal

Type of medication: NSAID

What it's used for: To ease arthritis pain and inflammation

Dosage: 500 to 1,500 mg per day in 2 doses

Special instructions: Do not take with other prescription or OTC NSAIDs. Take as directed at the same times every day. If you experience stomach upset, take with food, a glass of milk or an antacid.

Possible side effects: Abdominal or stomach cramps, pain or discomfort; diarrhea; dizziness; light-headedness; edema (swelling of feet); gastrointestinal bleeding; headache; heartburn or indigestion; nausea or vomiting; peptic ulcer

Be aware: Before taking this medication, let your doctor know if you drink alcohol or use blood thinners, or if you have or have had any of the following: sensitivity or allergy to aspirin or similar drugs, kidney or liver disease, heart disease, high blood pressure, asthma or stomach ulcers. Because stomach ulcers or internal bleeding can occur without warning, regular checkups are important. Patients on long-term NSAIDs should have blood counts and liver enzymes checked periodically.

Unlike low-dose aspirin, there is little evidence that this or other NSAIDs will protect against heart attack or stroke.

NSAIDs may be used with low-dose aspirin, but doing so may slightly increase your risk of gastric bleeding. Before taking this or any NSAID, tell your doctor if you take ACE inhibitors, lithium, warfarin or furosemide.

All NSAIDs may cause an increased risk of serious blood clots, heart attacks and stroke, which can be fatal. This risk may increase with dose and duration of use. Patients with cardiovascular disease or risk factors for cardiovascular disease may be at higher risk. These drugs should not be used for pain in people having coronary bypass surgery.

Dolacet

Generic name:
Hydrocodone with acetaminophen

Other brand name(s):
Hydrocet, Lorcet, Lortab, Vicodin

Type of medication: Analgesic

What it's used for: Pain not relieved by plain acetaminophen

Dosage: 2.5 to 10 mg hydrocodone every 4 to 6 hours as needed (Acetaminophen portion of medication varies.)

Special instructions: Do not increase dose on your own because side effects increase and tolerance develops as dosage increases; do not stop abruptly unless advised to do so by your doctor; do not drive or operate heavy machinery until you know how your body reacts to this drug.

Possible side effects: Constipation, dizziness, lightheadedness, mood changes, nausea, sedation, shortness of breath, vomiting and urinary retention

Be aware: If you consume 3 or more alcoholic drinks per day, consult your doctor before taking this medication. Mixing alcohol with acetaminophen can cause liver damage. Over time, this drug may cause psychological and physical dependence. Before taking this drug, let your doctor know if you use central nervous system depressants, such as antihistamines (allergy medications), tranquilizers, sleeping medications, muscle relaxants or narcotic pain medication, or if you have one of the following: liver disease, or history or alcohol or drug abuse. Avoid taking more than one product containing acetaminophen.

Duloxetine

Brand name(s):
Cymbalta

Type of medication: Antidepressant [selective serotonin and norepinephrine reuptake inhibitor (SSNRI)]

What it's used for: to improve depression, relieve fatigue and improve energy in people with fibromyalgia

Dosage: 60 mg twice daily

Special instructions: Build dose gradually; taper dose slowly.

Possible side effects: Anxiety or nervousness; constipation; decrease in sexual desire or ability; decreased appetite; diarrhea; drowsiness; dry mouth; headache; hives or itching; increased sweating; nausea; restlessness; skin rash; tiredness or weakness; trembling or shaking; trouble sleeping. Side effects may continue after treatment is stopped.

Be aware: Combining this drug with alcohol or other central nervous system depressants (including antihistamines, narcotic medications and some dental anesthetics) can increase their effects and side effects. Taking with aspirin or other NSAIDs may increase risk of bleeding. Never stop taking this medication abruptly. Your doctor will taper your dosage gradually. Do not take within 14 days of taking a monoamine oxidase (MAO) inhibitor. Patients and their family members should be aware of agitation and suicidal tendencies.

Ecotrin

Generic name:
Aspirin

Other brand name(s):
Anacin, Ascriptin, Bayer, Bufferin, Excedrin tablets

Type of medication: NSAID, salicylate (OTC)

What it's used for: To ease pain and inflammation associated with many forms of arthritis

Dosage: 2,400 to 5,400 mg per day in several doses

Special instructions: Take with food. Do not chew tablets; do not crush enteric-coated or time-release forms and mix with water. Do not combine with other NSAIDs.

Possible side effects: Abdominal or stomach cramps, pain or discomfort; diarrhea; dizziness, drowsiness or light-headedness; edema (swelling of the feet); headache; heartburn or indigestion; nausea or vomiting

Be aware: Ulcers and internal bleeding can occur without warning, so regular checkups are important. Confusion, deafness, dizziness or ringing in the ears indicates you are taking too much. Before taking this drug, let your doctor know if you drink alcohol, use blood thinners or have any of the following: sensitivity or allergy to aspirin or similar drugs, kidney disease, liver disease, asthma or peptic ulcers. If you are taking doses of more than 3,600 mg per day, your doctor should monitor the salicylate levels in your blood.

Enbrel

Generic name:
Etanercept

Type of medication: Biologic response modifier

What it's used for: To ease symptoms, prevent joint damage and improve physical function in people with moderately to severely active rheumatoid arthritis; to reduce signs and symptoms of polyarticular juvenile rheumatoid arthritis; to ease symptoms and stop joint damage in psoriatic arthritis, to ease symptoms of ankylosing spondylitis and to treat severe plaque psoriasis.

Dosage: For adults with RA, psoriatic arthritis or ankylosing spondylitis, the recommended dose of *Enbrel* is 50 mg given once per week by one subcutaneous (beneath the skin) injection. The usual starting dose of *Enbrel* is 50-mg injections twice weekly for three months. Starting doses of 25 mg or 50 mg per week were also efficacious.

Special instructions: *Enbrel* single-use prefilled syringes must be refrigerated. Before injection, the prefilled syringe may be allowed to reach room temperature (approximately 15 to 30 minutes). The needle cover should not be removed while allowing the prefilled syringe to reach room temperature.

Possible side effects: Redness and pain, itching, swelling and/or bruising at the injection site; upper respiratory infection

Be aware: Rheumatoid arthritis carries a higher risk of infection and lymphoma. It is uncertain whether this and other biologic response modifiers increase lymphoma risk. This agent should be discontinued if you have a serious or recurrent infection (such as pneumonia). Live vaccine should not be given along with this drug, but the flu or pneumonia vaccine (*Pneumovax*) can be safely given.

Let your doctor know if you have a history of (or currently have) one of the following: active infection, recurrent infection, exposure to tuberculosis or positive skin test for tuberculosis; or if you have a nervous system disorder, including neurological disorders such as multiple sclerosis, seizure disorders, myelitis or optic neuritis.

Rarely a lupus-like syndrome may develop, with symptoms such as rash, fever and pleurisy, which may resolve when medication is stopped. Multiple sclerosis has rarely developed in patients receiving this or infliximab. Seizures have been reported with this drug. *Enbrel* should be used with caution in patients with congestive heart failure (CHF).

Endep

Generic name:
Amitriptyline hydrochloride

Other brand name(s):
Elavil

Type of medication: Antidepressant (tricyclic)

What it's used for: To relieve pain and promote sleep in fibromyalgia

Dosage: 10 to 80 mg per day in a single dose

Special instructions: Take at bedtime or several hours before bedtime to avoid "morning hangover."

Possible side effects: Constipation, dizziness, drowsiness, dry mouth, headache, fatigue, weight gain

Be aware: Before taking this medication, tell your doctor if you are using another antidepressant or have any of the following: a history of seizures, urinary retention, heart problems, or glaucoma or other chronic eye condition. Because adverse side effects can occur if you stop using this drug abruptly, discontinue it gradually. Know how you respond to this drug before driving or operating heavy machinery.

Endocet

Generic name:
oxycodone with acetaminophen

Other brand names:
Percocet

Type of medication: analgesic

What it's used for: severe pain from arthritis, surgery or fractures

Dosage: 5 mg oxycodone every 6 hours as needed (Acetaminophen portion of medication varies, depending on whether you are taking pills or capsules.)

Special instructions: Never chew or cut tablets; a potentially fatal dose can occur if the medication is released rapidly. Must be taken whole.

Possible side effects: Constipation, dizziness, drowsiness, dry mouth, headache, increased sweating, itching of skin, nausea, shortness of breath, vomiting, weakness

Be aware: If you consume 3 or more alcoholic drinks per day, consult your doctor before taking this medication. Mixing acetaminophen with alcohol can cause liver damage.

Over time this drug may cause psychological and physical dependence. Before taking this drug, let your doctor know if you use a central nervous system depressant, such as antihistamines (allergy medications), tranquilizers, sleeping medications, narcotic pain medications or if you have one of the following: liver disease, or history of alcohol or drug abuse.

Estrogens

Brand name(s):
With progesterone: Premphase, Prempro, Activella
Estratab, Estrace, Menest
Without progesterone: Premarin

Type of medication: Hormone

What it's used for: To prevent and treat osteoporosis

Dosage: 0.625 mg per day continuously in 28-day cycles (progesterone component of drug varies depending on day of cycle) (*Premphase, Prempro, Activella*); 0.3 mg to 0.6 mg per day in a single dose (*Estratab, Estrace, Meneset*); 1 mg estradiol patch delivers 14 mcg estradiol per day for 7 days (*Menostar*)

Special instructions: Apply patches to clean, dry skin of lower abdomen.

Possible side effects: Bloating of stomach; breast pain; increased breast size; nausea; swelling of feet and lower legs; weight gain. Increased risk of breast cancer and cardiovascular disease

Be aware: Women who have not had a hysterectomy should take estrogen in conjunction with progesterone. Before taking this drug, consult with your doctor about the possible risk of heart disease, breast or uterine cancer, blood clots and other side effects. Let your doctor know if you have liver dysfunction or disease or hypersensitivity to the medication's ingredients. Estrogens should not be used for prevention of cardiovascular disease or dementia.

Estratab, see Estrogens

Estrace, see Estrogens

Etanercept

Brand name(s):
Enbrel

Type of medication: Biologic response modifier

What it's used for: To ease symptoms, prevent joint damage and improve physical function in people with moderately to severely active rheumatoid arthritis; to reduce signs and symptoms of polyarticular juvenile rheumatoid arthritis; to ease symptoms and stop joint damage in psoriatic arthritis; to ease symptoms of ankylosing spondylitis and to treat severe plaque psoriasis.

Dosage: For adults with RA, psoriatic arthritis or ankylosing spondylitis, the recommended dose of etanercept is 50 mg given once per week by one subcutaneous (beneath the skin) injection. The usual starting dose of etanercept is 50-mg injections twice weekly for three months. Starting doses of 25 mg or 50 mg per week were also efficacious.

Special instructions: *Enbrel* single-use prefilled syringes must be refrigerated. Before injection, the prefilled syringe may be allowed to reach room temperature (approximately 15 to 30 minutes). The needle cover should not be removed while allowing the prefilled syringe to reach room temperature.

Possible side effects: Redness and pain, itching, swelling and/or bruising at the injection site; upper respiratory infection

Be aware: Rheumatoid arthritis carries a higher risk of infection and lymphoma. It is uncertain whether this and other biologic response modifiers increase lymphoma risk. This agent should be discontinued if you have a serious or recurrent infection (such as pneumonia). Live vaccine should not be given along with this drug, but the flu or pneumonia vaccine (*Pneumovax*) can be safely given.

Let your doctor know if you have a history of (or currently have) one of the following: active infection, recurrent infection, exposure to tuberculosis or positive skin test for tuberculosis; or if you have a nervous system disorder, including neurological disorders such as multiple sclerosis, seizure disorders, myelitis or optic neuritis.

Rarely a lupus-like syndrome may develop, with symptoms such as rash, fever and pleurisy, which may resolve when medication is stopped. Multiple sclerosis has rarely developed in patients receiving this or infliximab. Seizures have been reported with this drug. Etanercept should be used with caution in patients with congestive heart failure (CHF).

Etodolac

Brand name(s):
Lodine, Lodine XL

Type of medication: NSAID

What it's used for: To ease arthritis pain and inflammation

Dosage: 600 to 1,200 mg per day in 2 or 3 doses (*Lodine*); 600 mg per day in a single dose (*Lodine XL*)

Special instructions: Do not take with other prescription or OTC NSAIDs. Take as directed at the same times every day. If you experience stomach upset, take with food, a glass of milk or an antacid.

Possible side effects: Abdominal or stomach cramps, pain or discomfort; diarrhea; dizziness; light-headedness; edema (swelling of feet); gastrointestinal bleeding; headache; heartburn or indigestion; nausea or vomiting; peptic ulcer

Be aware: Before taking this medication, let your doctor know if you drink alcohol or use blood thinners or if you have or have had any of the following: sensitivity or allergy to aspirin or similar drugs, kidney or liver disease, heart disease, high blood pressure, asthma or stomach ulcers. Because stomach ulcers or internal bleeding can occur without warning, regular checkups are important. Patients on long-term NSAIDs should have blood counts and liver enzymes checked periodically.

Unlike low-dose aspirin, there is little evidence that this or other NSAIDs will protect against heart attack or stroke. NSAIDs may be used with low-dose aspirin, but doing so may slightly increase your risk of gastric bleeding. Before taking this or any NSAID, tell your doctor if you take ACE inhibitors, lithium, warfarin or furosemide.

All NSAIDs may cause an increased risk of serious blood clots, heart attacks and stroke, which can be fatal. This risk may increase with dose and duration of use. Patients with cardiovascular disease or risk factors for cardiovascular disease may be at higher risk. These drugs should not be used for pain in people having coronary bypass surgery.

Evista

Generic name:
Raloxifene hydrochloride

Type of medication: Selective estrogen receptor molecule (SERM)

What it's used for: Osteoporosis

Dosage: 60 mg per day in a single dose

Possible side effects: Blood clots in veins, hot flashes, leg cramps

Be aware: This drug should not be used prior to menopause. Let your doctor know if there is a chance you could be pregnant or if you have a history of blood clots, or if you use cholestyramine or warfarin (*Coumadin*).

Evoxac

Generic name (s):
Civemeline

Type of medication: Cholinergic agonist

What it's used for: To increase saliva production, relieve dry mouth associated with Sjögren's syndrome

Dosage: 30 mg three times per day

Special instructions: Start with a low dose and take after meals to minimize side effects. Allow 6 to 12 weeks of uninterrupted treatment before treatment is noticed.

Possible side effects: Changes in heart rate (rare); diarrhea; excessive sweating; nausea; problems with night vision; rhinitis

Be aware: Do not take if you have uncontrolled asthma, chronic bronchitis, chronic obstructive pulmonary disease, significant cardiovascular disease, acute iritis or narrow-angle glaucoma. Let your doctor know if you take beta-adrenergic antagonists (beta blockers).

Excedrin caplets

Generic name:
Acetaminophen

Other brand name(s):
Anacin (aspirin-free), Panadol, Tylenol,
Tylenol Arthritis Pain

Type of Medication: Analgesic (OTC)

What it's used for: To relieve pain in any form of arthritis

Dosage: 325 to 1,000 mg every 4 to 6 hours as needed, no more than 4,000 mg per day

Special instructions: Do not use with any other product containing acetaminophen; do not use for more than 10 days for pain – unless directed by a doctor.

Possible side effects: When taken as directed, acetaminophen is usually not associated with side effects.

Be aware: If you consume 3 or more alcoholic drinks per day, consult your doctor before taking acetaminophen. This medication can cause liver damage. Mixing acetaminophen with alcohol can cause liver damage.

Excedrin tablets

Generic name:
Aspirin

Other brand name(s):
Anacin, Ascriptin, Bayer, Bufferin, Ecotrin

Type of medication: NSAIDs, salicylate (OTC)

What it's used for: To ease pain and inflammation associated with many forms of arthritis

Dosage: 2,400 to 5,400 mg per day in several doses

Special instructions: Take with food. Do not chew tablets; do not crush enteric-coated or time-release forms and mix with water. Do not combine with other NSAIDs.

Possible side effects: Abdominal or stomach cramps, pain or discomfort; diarrhea; dizziness, drowsiness or light-headedness; edema (swelling of the feet); headache; heartburn or indigestion; nausea or vomiting

Be aware: Ulcers and internal bleeding can occur without warning, so regular checkups are important. Confusion, deafness, dizziness or ringing in the ears indicates you are taking too much. Before taking this drug, let your doctor know if you drink alcohol, use blood thinners or have any of the following: sensitivity or allergy to aspirin or similar drugs, kidney disease, liver disease, asthma or peptic ulcers. If you are taking doses of more than 3,600 mg per day, your doctor should monitor the salicylate levels in your blood.

Feldene

Generic name:
Piroxicam

Type of medication: NSAID

What it's used for: To ease arthritis pain and inflammation

Dosage: 20 mg per day in 1 or 2 doses

Special instructions: Do not take with other prescription or OTC NSAIDs. Take as directed at the same time(s) every day. If you experience stomach upset, take with food, a glass of milk or an antacid.

Possible side effects: Abdominal or stomach cramps, pain or discomfort; diarrhea; dizziness; edema (swelling of the feet); gastrointestinal bleeding; headache; heartburn or indigestion; nausea or vomiting; peptic ulcer

Be aware: Before taking this medication, let your doctor know if you drink alcohol or use blood thinners, or if you have or have had any of the following: sensitivity or allergy to aspirin or similar drugs, kidney or liver disease, heart disease, high blood pressure, asthma or stomach ulcers. Because stomach ulcers or internal bleeding can occur without warning, regular checkups are important. Patients on long-term NSAIDs should have blood counts and liver enzymes checked periodically.

Unlike low-dose aspirin, there is little evidence that this or other NSAIDs will protect against heart attack or stroke.

NSAIDs may be used with low-dose aspirin, but doing so may slightly increase your risk of gastric bleeding. Before taking this or any NSAID, tell your doctor if you take ACE inhibitors, lithium, warfarin or furosemide.

All NSAIDs may cause an increased risk of serious blood clots, heart attacks and stroke, which can be fatal. This risk may increase with dose and duration of use. Patients with cardiovascular disease or risk factors for cardiovascular disease may be at higher risk. These drugs should not be used for pain in people having coronary bypass surgery.

Fenoprofen calcium

Brand name(s):
Nalfon

Type of medication: NSAID

What it's used for: To ease arthritis pain and inflammation

Dosage: 900 to 2,400 mg per day in 3 or 4 doses; never more than 3,200 mg per day

Special instructions: Do not take with other prescription or OTC NSAIDs. Take as directed at the same time(s) every day. If you experience stomach upset, take with food or a glass of milk.

Possible side effects: Abdominal or stomach cramps, pain or discomfort; diarrhea; dizziness; edema (swelling of the feet); gastrointestinal bleeding; headache; heartburn or indigestion; nausea or vomiting; peptic ulcer

Be aware: Before taking this medication, let your doctor know if you drink alcohol or use blood thinners or if you have or have had any of the following: sensitivity or allergy to aspirin or similar drugs, kidney or liver disease, heart disease, high blood pressure, asthma or stomach ulcers. Because stomach ulcers or internal bleeding can occur without warning, regular checkups are important. Patients on long-term NSAIDs should have blood counts and liver enzymes checked periodically.

Unlike low-dose aspirin, there is little evidence that this or other NSAIDs will protect against heart attack or stroke. NSAIDs may be used with low-dose aspirin, but doing so may slightly increase your risk of gastric bleeding. Before taking this or any NSAID, tell your doctor if you take ACE inhibitors, lithium, warfarin or furosemide.

All NSAIDs may cause an increased risk of serious blood clots, heart attacks and stroke, which can be fatal. This risk may increase with dose and duration of use. Patients with cardiovascular disease or risk factors for cardiovascular disease may be at higher risk. These drugs should not be used for pain in people having coronary bypass surgery.

Flexeril

Generic name:
Cyclobenzaprine

Other brand name(s):
Cycloflex

Type of medication: Muscle relaxant

What it's used for: To promote sleep and ease muscle pain in fibromyalgia

Dosage: 5 to 30 mg per day in a single dose

Special instructions: Take 2 to 3 hours before bedtime to reduce "morning hangover."

Possible side effects: Blurred vision; dizziness or light-headedness; drowsiness; dry mouth

Be aware: Before taking this medication, let your doctor know if you use alcohol or other central nervous system (CNS) depressants such as antihistamines, cold or allergy medications, tranquilizers, sleeping medications, muscle relaxants or narcotic pain medication, or if you have any of the following: glaucoma, problems with urination, heart or blood vessel disease or overactive thyroid.

Fluoxetine

Brand name(s):
Prozac

Type of medication: Antidepressant (SSRI)

What it's used for: To improve depression, relieve fatigue and improve energy in people with fibromyalgia

Dosage: 20 to 80 mg per day in a single dose

Special instructions: Build dose gradually; taper dose slowly.

Possible side effects: Anxiety or nervousness; constipation; decrease in sexual desire or ability; decreased appetite; diarrhea; drowsiness; dry mouth; headache; hives or itching; increased sweating; nausea; restlessness; skin rash; tiredness or weakness; trembling or shaking; trouble sleeping. Side effects may continue after treatment is stopped.

Be aware: Combining this drug with alcohol or other central nervous system depressants (including antihistamines, narcotic medications and some dental anesthetics) can increase their effects and side effects. Taking with aspirin or other NSAIDs may increase risk of bleeding. Never stop taking this medication abruptly. Your doctor will taper your dosage gradually. Do not take within 14 days of taking a monoamine oxidase (MAO) inhibitor. Patients and their family members should be aware of agitation and suicidal tendencies.

Flurbiprofen

Brand name(s):
Ansaid

Type of medication: NSAID

What it's used for: To ease arthritis pain and inflammation

Dosage: 200 to 300 mg per day in 2 to 4 doses

Special instructions: Do not take with other prescription or OTC NSAIDs. Take as directed at the same time(s) every day. If you experience stomach upset, take with food, a glass of milk or an antacid.

Possible side effects: Abdominal or stomach cramps, pain or discomfort; diarrhea; dizziness; edema (swelling of the feet); gastrointestinal bleeding; headache; heartburn or indigestion; nausea or vomiting; peptic ulcer

Be aware: Before taking this medication, let your doctor know if you drink alcohol or use blood thinners or if you have or have had any of the following: sensitivity or allergy to aspirin or similar drugs, kidney or liver disease, heart disease, high blood pressure, asthma or stomach ulcers. Because stomach ulcers or internal bleeding can occur without warning, regular checkups are important. Patients on long-term NSAIDs should have blood counts and liver enzymes checked periodically.

Unlike low-dose aspirin, there is little evidence that this or other NSAIDs will protect against heart attack or stroke.

NSAIDs may be used with low-dose aspirin, but doing so may slightly increase your risk of gastric bleeding. Before taking this or any NSAID, tell your doctor if you take ACE inhibitors, lithium, warfarin or furosemide.

All NSAIDs may cause an increased risk of serious blood clots, heart attacks and stroke, which can be fatal. This risk may increase with dose and duration of use. Patients with cardiovascular disease or risk factors for cardiovascular disease may be at higher risk. These drugs should not be used for pain in people having coronary bypass surgery.

Forteo

Generic name:
Teriparatide

Type of medication: Bone formation agent

What it's used for: Osteoporosis

Dosage: 20 micrograms (mcg) per day in a single dose

Special instructions: Inject into the abdomen or thigh using a multidose prefilled pen delivery device provided by the manufacturer.

Possible side effects: Dizziness, leg cramps

Be aware: Do not take this drug if you have ever had cancer of the bone or radiation therapy for bone or if you have high blood levels of calcium. Urinary excretion of calcium should be monitored if you have urinary tract stones or a high calcium level.

Fosamax

Generic name:
Alendronate

Type of medication: Bisphosphonate

What it's used for: To prevent or treat osteoporosis

Dosage: For corticosteroid-induced osteoporosis: 5 mg per day in a single dose (10 mg if postmenopausal); for general osteoporosis treatment: 10 mg per day in a single dose or 70 mg per week in a single dose; For osteoporosis prevention: 5 mg per day in a single dose or 35 mg per week in a single dose

Special instructions: Take with a full glass (8 ounces) of water first thing in the morning. Do not eat or drink anything else or take any other medication, including calcium tablets, for at least 30 minutes after taking the drug. Stay upright (sitting or standing) for at least 30 minutes after taking the drug to avoid irritating the esophagus.

Possible side effects: Abdominal or stomach pain; heartburn

Be aware: Before taking this medication, let your doctor know if you have problems with the esophagus, stomach or kidneys. Blood levels of calcium and vitamin D must be normal before starting therapy.

Fosamax Plus D

Generic name(s):

Alendronate with vitamin D

Type of medication: Bisphosphonate with vitamin D supplement

What it's used for: To treat osteoporosis

Dosage: Single dose of 70 mg alendronate and 2,800 IUs vitamin D

Special instructions: Take with a full glass (8 ounces) of water first thing in the morning. Do not eat or drink anything else or take any other medication, including calcium tablets, for at least 30 minutes after taking the drug. Take medication while sitting or standing and stay upright for at least 30 minutes to avoid irritating the esophagus.

Possible side effects: Abdominal or stomach pain; heartburn

Be aware: Before taking this medication, let your doctor know if you have problems with the esophagus, stomach or kidneys. Blood levels of calcium and vitamin D must be normal before starting therapy.

Gold, oral – auranofin

Brand name(s):

Ridaura

Type of medication: DMARD

What it's used for: Rheumatoid arthritis

Dosage: 6 to 9 mg per day in 1 or 2 doses

Special instructions: Take with a glass of milk or water. If stomach upset occurs, take with food.

Possible side effects: Diarrhea, low blood counts, metallic taste in mouth, mouth ulcers, protein in urine, skin rash or itching

Be aware: Before taking this drug, let your doctor know if you have or have had one of the following: adverse reaction to a gold-containing medication, a history of blood-cell abnormality, inflammatory bowel disease, or kidney or liver disease. This drug can cause sun sensitivity, so minimize exposure to sunlight and sunlamps and wear sunscreen. Your doctor should order periodic blood and urine tests to check for effects on the blood and kidneys.

Gold, injectable, see Gold sodium thiomalate

Gold sodium thiomalate (Injectable gold)

Brand name(s):
Myochrysine

Type of medication: DMARD

What it's used for: Rheumatoid arthritis

Dosage: 10 mg the first week, then 25 to 50 mg per week thereafter. Frequency may be reduced after several months.

Possible side effects: Irritation and soreness of tongue; irritated or bleeding gums; metallic taste; skin rash or itching; ulcers, sores or white spots on lips or in mouth or throat

Be aware: Before taking this medication, let your doctor know if you have any of the following: lupus, skin rash, kidney disease or colitis. Increased joint pain may occur for one or two days after injection, but it usually disappears after the first few injections. Your doctor should order periodic urine and blood tests to check for side effects.

Hexadrol

Generic name:
Dexamethasone

Other brand name(s):
Decadron

Type of medication: Corticosteroid

What it's used for: To control inflammation of joints and organs in many forms of arthritis and related conditions

Dosage: Dosage varies widely according to the disease being treated. Taking either too much or too little can be dangerous. Take exactly the amount prescribed by your doctor.

Special instructions: Take with food. A single daily dose should be taken with breakfast. Sometimes the dose is split, taken 2 to 4 times per day. Don't stop medication abruptly; dosage must be tapered or reduced gradually.

Possible side effects: Bruising, cataracts, elevated blood fats (cholesterol, triglycerides), elevated blood sugar, hardening of the arteries (atherosclerosis), hypertension, increased appetite, indigestion, insomnia, mood swings, muscle weakness, nervousness or restlessness, osteoporosis, susceptibility to infection, thin skin

Be aware: Before taking this medication, let your doctor know if you have one of the following: fungal infection, history of tuberculosis, underactive thyroid, diabetes, stomach ulcer, high blood pressure or osteoporosis.

Humira

Generic name:
Adalimumab

Type of medication: Biologic response modifier

What it's used for: To ease RA symptoms, prevent joint damage and improve physical function in adults with moderately to severely active RA.

Dosage: 40 mg once every two weeks when given with methrotrexate. Some patients not also taking methotrexate may benefit from taking 40 mg weekly.

Special instructions: Drug must be refrigerated but not

frozen prior to use. Comes in prefilled syringes and may be injected into the thigh, abdomen or upper arm.

Possible side effects: Redness and pain, itching, swelling and/or bruising at the injection site; upper respiratory infection

Be aware: Rheumatoid arthritis carries a higher risk of infection and lymphoma. It is uncertain whether this and other biologic response modifiers increase lymphoma risk. This agent should be discontinued if you have a serious infection or recurrent infections (such as pneumonia). Live vaccine should not be given along with this drug, but the pneumonia vaccine (*Pneumovax*) can be safely given.

Let your doctor know if you have a history of (or currently have) one of the following: active infection, recurrent infection, exposure to tuberculosis or positive skin test for tuberculosis; or if you have a nervous system disorder, including neurological disorders such as multiple sclerosis, seizure disorders, myelitis or optic neuritis.

Patients with congestive heart failure (CHF) should not be given this drug.

Hydrocet, see hydrocodone with acetaminophen

Hydrocodone with acetaminophen

Brand name(s):
Dolacet, Hydrocet, Lorcet, Lortab, Vicodin

Type of medication: Analgesic

What it's used for: Pain not relieved by plain acetaminophen

Dosage: 2.5 to 10 mg hydrocodone every 4 to 6 hours as needed. (Acetaminophen portion of medication varies.)

Special instructions: Do not increase dose on your own because side effects increase and tolerance develops as dosage increases; do not stop abruptly unless advised to do so by your doctor; do not drive or operate heavy machinery until you know how your body reacts to this drug.

Possible side effects: Constipation, dizziness, lightheadedness, mood changes, nausea, sedation, shortness of breath, vomiting and urinary retention

Be aware: If you consume 3 or more alcoholic drinks per day, consult your doctor before taking acetaminophen. Mixing acetaminophen with alcohol can cause liver damage. Over time, this drug may cause psychological and physical dependence. Before taking this drug, let your doctor know if you use central nervous system depressants, such as antihistamines (allergy medications), tranquilizers, sleeping medications, muscle relaxants or narcotic pain medication, or if you have one of the following: liver disease, or history or alcohol or drug abuse.

Hydrocortisone

Brand name(s):
Cortef, Hydrocortone

Type of medication: Corticosteroid

What it's used for: To control inflammation of joints and organs in many forms of arthritis and related conditions

Dosage: Dosage varies widely according to the disease being treated. Taking either too much or too little can be dangerous. Take exactly the amount prescribed by your doctor.

Special instructions: Take with food. A single daily dose should be taken with breakfast. Sometimes the dose is split, taken 2 to 4 times per day. Don't stop medication abruptly; dosage must be tapered or reduced gradually.

Possible side effects: Bruising, cataracts, elevated blood fats (cholesterol, triglycerides), elevated blood sugar, hardening of the arteries (atherosclerosis), hypertension, increased appetite, indigestion, insomnia, mood swings, muscle weakness, nervousness or restlessness, osteoporosis, susceptibility to infection, thin skin

Be aware: Before taking this medication, let your doctor know if you have one of the following: fungal infection, history of tuberculosis, underactive thyroid, diabetes, stomach ulcer, high blood pressure or osteoporosis.

Hydrocortone, see hydrocortisone

Hydroxychloroquine sulfate

Brand name(s):
Plaquenil

Type of medication: DMARD

What it's used for: Rheumatoid arthritis, lupus

Dosage: 200 to 600 mg per day in 1 or 2 doses

Possible side effects: Blurred vision; diarrhea; headache; increased sensitivity to sunlight; itching; loss of appetite; nausea or vomiting; rashes; stomach cramps or pain

Be aware: Before taking this medication, let your doctor know if you have any eye problems, including a retinal abnormality. Because vision may be damaged with long-term therapy (given over several years), you may need to have an eye exam when you start taking the drug and every 6 to 12 months thereafter to detect retinal changes.

Hydroxypropyl cellulose pellets

Brand name(s):
Lacrisert

Type of medication: Artificial tears

What it's used for: To relieve dry eyes associated with Sjögren's syndrome

Dosage: 1 pellet in lower lids twice per day

Special instructions: Small pellets are placed in lower eyelid. Adding artificial tears makes pellet dissolve, creating and locking in moisture

Possible side effects: Eye pain; irritation or redness of eye; vision changes

Ibandronate

Brand name:
Boniva

Type of medication: Bisphosphonate

What it's used for: Postmenopausal osteoporosis

Dosage: 150 mg taken as a single monthly dose

Special instructions: Take only with one cup of water first thing in the morning. Swallow pill whole while sitting or standing; stay upright and avoid food for 60 minutes.

Possible side effects: Abdominal or stomach pain; heartburn

Be aware: Before taking this medication, tell your doctor if you are taking aspirin or aspirin-containing products, or if you have problems with the esophagus, stomach or kidneys. Blood levels of calcium and vitamin D must be normal before starting therapy.

Ibuprofen

Brand name(s):
Prescription: Motrin
Non-prescription: Advil, Motrin IB, Nuprin

Type of medication: NSAID

What it's used for: To ease arthritis pain and inflammation

Dosage: 1,200 to 3,000 mg per day in 3 or 4 doses (prescription); 200 to 400 mg every 4 to 6 hours as needed, no more than 1,200 mg per day (OTC)

Special instructions: Do not take with other prescription or OTC NSAIDs. Take as directed at the same time(s) every day. If stomach upset occurs, take with food or a glass of milk.

Possible side effects: Abdominal or stomach cramps, pain or discomfort; diarrhea; dizziness; edema (swelling of the feet); gastrointestinal bleeding; headache; heartburn or indigestion; nausea or vomiting; peptic ulcer

Be aware: Before taking this medication, let your doctor know if you drink alcohol or use blood thinners, or if you have or have had any of the following: sensitivity or allergy to aspirin or similar drugs, kidney or liver disease, heart disease, high blood pressure, asthma or stomach ulcers. Because stomach ulcers or internal bleeding can occur without warning, regular checkups are important. Patients on long-term NSAIDs should have blood counts and liver enzymes checked periodically.

Unlike low-dose aspirin, there is little evidence that this drug or other NSAIDs will protect against heart attack or stroke. NSAIDs may be used with low-dose aspirin, but doing so may slightly increase your risk of gastric bleeding. Before taking this or any NSAID, tell your doctor if you take ACE inhibitors, lithium, warfarin or furosemide.

All NSAIDs may cause an increased risk of serious blood clots, heart attacks and stroke, which can be fatal. This risk may increase with dose and duration of use. Patients with cardiovascular disease or risk factors for cardiovascular disease may be at higher risk. These drugs should not be used for pain in people having coronary bypass surgery.

Imuran

Generic name:
Azathioprine

Type of medication: DMARD

What it's used for: Rheumatoid arthritis, lupus and other autoimmune diseases

Dosage: 50 to 150 mg per day in 1 to 3 doses

Special instructions: Take with food.

Possible side effects: Fever or chills, loss of appetite, liver problems, low blood counts, nausea or vomiting, unusual tiredness or weakness

Be aware: Before taking this drug, tell your doctor if you use allopurinol or have kidney or liver disease. This drug can be associated with developments of certain cancers such as lymphoma. Your doctor may order periodic blood tests to check for effects on the blood.

Indocin, see **Indomethacin**

Indocin SR, see **Indomethacin**

Indomethacin

Brand name(s):
Indocin, Indocin SR

Type of medication: NSAID

What it's used for: To ease arthritis pain and inflammation

Dosage: 50 to 200 mg per day in 2 to 4 doses (*Indocin*); 75 mg per day in a single dose or 150 mg per day in 2 doses (*Indocin SR*)

Special instructions: Do not take with other prescription or OTC NSAIDs. Take as directed at the same time(s) every day. If you experience stomach upset, take with food, a glass of milk or an antacid.

Possible side effects: Abdominal or stomach cramps, pain or discomfort; diarrhea; dizziness; edema (swelling of the feet); headache; gastrointestinal bleeding; heartburn or indigestion; nausea or vomiting; peptic ulcer

Be aware: Before taking this medication, let your doctor know if you drink alcohol or use blood thinners or if you have or have had any of the following: sensitivity or allergy to aspirin or similar drugs, kidney or liver disease, heart disease, high blood pressure, asthma or stomach ulcers. Because stomach ulcers or internal bleeding can occur without warning, regular checkups are important. Patients on long-term NSAIDs should have blood counts and liver enzymes checked periodically.

Unlike low-dose aspirin, there is little evidence that this or other NSAIDs will protect against heart attack or stroke. NSAIDs may be used with low-dose aspirin, but doing so may slightly increase your risk of gastric bleeding. Before taking this or any NSAID, tell your doctor if you take ACE inhibitors, lithium, warfarin or furosemide.

All NSAIDs may cause an increased risk of serious blood clots, heart attacks and stroke, which can be fatal. This risk may increase with dose and duration of use. Patients with cardiovascular disease or risk factors for cardiovascular disease may be at higher risk. These drugs should not be used for pain in people having coronary bypass surgery.

Infliximab

Brand name(s):
Remicade

Type of medication: Biologic response modifier

What it's used for: To control symptoms, prevent joint damage and improve physical function in rheumatoid arthritis, psoriatic arthritis and ankylosing spondylitis.

Dosage: Dose is based on body weight and ranges from 200 mg to 400 mg per treatment for most patients. After three initial infusions at 0, 2 and 6 weeks, infusions are repeated every 8 weeks.

Special instructions: Drug is infused intravenously (IV) during a 2-hour infusion done in a doctor's office, clinic or hospital. Patients taking infliximab should also be taking methotrexate once a week by mouth or injection.

Possible side effects: Infusion reactions (occurring during or shortly after the infusion) including chest pain, change in blood pressure, difficulty breathing and hives; upper respiratory infection; redness and pain; itching, swelling and/or bruising at the injection site

Be aware: Rheumatoid arthritis carries a higher risk of infection and lymphoma. It is uncertain whether this and other biologic response modifiers increase lymphoma risk. Discontinue if you have a serious infection (such as pneumonia) or recurrent infections. Live vaccines should not be given along with this drug, but the vaccine for pneumonia (*Pneumovax*) can be safely given.

Let your doctor know if you have a history of (or currently have) one of the following: active infection, recurrent infection, exposure to tuberculosis or positive skin test for tuberculosis; or if you have a nervous system disorder, including neurological disorders such as multiple sclerosis, seizure disorders, myelitis or optic neuritis.

Patients with congestive heart failure (CHF) should not be given this drug.

Rare reports of lupus may develop with symptoms such as rash, fever and pleurisy. These symptoms may resolve when the medication is stopped. Multiple sclerosis has rarely developed in patients receiving this drug or etanercept.

Infusion reaction may be treated by slowing the speed of infusion as well as by pre-treatment with acetaminophen, antihistamine (*Benadryl, Claritin*) or steroid medication (hydrocortisone, prednisone).

Ketoprofen

Brand name(s):

Prescription: Orudis, Oruvail
Non-prescription: Actron, Orudis KT

Type of medication: NSAID

What it's used for: To ease arthritis pain and inflammation

Dosage: 200 to 225 mg per day in 3 or 4 doses (*Orudis*); 150 or 200 mg per day in a single dose (*Oruvail*); 12.5 mg every 4 to 6 hours as needed (non-prescription brands)

Special instructions: Do not take with other prescription or OTC NSAIDs. Take as directed at the same time(s) every day. If you experience stomach upset, take with food, a glass of milk or an antacid.

Possible side effects: Abdominal or stomach cramps, pain or discomfort; edema (swelling of the feet); diarrhea; dizziness; gastrointestinal bleeding; headache; heartburn or indigestion; nausea or vomiting; peptic ulcer

Be aware: Before taking this medication, let your doctor know if you drink alcohol or use blood thinners, or if you have or have had any of the following: sensitivity or allergy to aspirin or similar drugs, kidney or liver disease, heart disease, high blood pressure, asthma or stomach ulcers. Because stomach ulcers or internal bleeding can occur without warning, regular checkups are important. Patients on long-term NSAIDs should have blood counts and liver enzymes checked periodically.

Unlike low-dose aspirin, there is little evidence that this or other NSAIDs will protect against heart attack or stroke. NSAIDs may be used with low dose aspirin, but doing so may slightly increase your risk of gastric bleeding. Before taking this or any NSAID, tell your doctor if you take ACE inhibitors, lithium, warfarin or furosemide.

All NSAIDs may cause an increased risk of serious blood clots, heart attacks and stroke, which can be fatal. This risk may increase with dose and duration of use. Patients with cardiovascular disease or risk factors for cardiovascular disease may be at higher risk. These drugs should not be used for pain in people having coronary bypass surgery.

Kineret

Generic name:
Anakinra

Type of medication: Biologic response modifier

What it's used for: To ease symptoms of rheumatoid arthritis and prevent joint damage

Dosage: 100 mg given once daily by subcutaneous (beneath the skin) injection; 100 mg every other day for patients with severe kidney disease

Special instructions: Refrigerate prior to use. Prefilled syringes can be self-injected with or without the aid of an automatic injector device (*SimpleJect*) available through the manufacturer. Do not shake. May be injected into the thigh, abdomen or upper arm. Try to administer at the same time every day.

Possible side effects: Injection site reactions (usually occurring during the first 4 to 6 weeks of use), including redness, swelling, pain and bruising; low white blood cell or platelet count; upper respiratory infection

Be aware: Rheumatoid arthritis carries a higher risk of infection and lymphoma. It is uncertain whether this and other biologic response modifiers increase lymphoma risk. Discontinue if you have a serious infection (such as pneumonia) or recurrent infections. Live vaccine should not be given along with this drug, but the vaccine for pneumonia (*Pneumovax*) can be safely given.

Serious infections, such as pneumonia, occur in approximately 2 percent of people taking this drug. Inform your doctor if you have a current infection or history of serious infection.

Lacrisert

Generic name:
Hydroxypropyl cellulose pellets

Type of medication: Artificial tears

What it's used for: To relieve dry eyes associated with Sjögren's syndrome

Dosage: 1 pellet in lower lids twice per day

Special instructions: Small pellets are placed in lower eyelid. Adding artificial tears makes pellet dissolve, creating and locking in moisture

Possible side effects: Eye pain; irritation or redness of eye; vision changes

Leflunomide

Brand name(s):
Arava

Type of medication: DMARD

What it's used for: Rheumatoid arthritis

Dosage: 10 to 20 mg per day in a single dose

Possible side effects: Dizziness, gastrointestinal problems, hair loss, headache, heartburn, high blood pressure, liver problems, low blood cell count, pain or burning in feet or hands (neuropathy) skin rash, stomach pain, sneezing, sore throat

Be aware: Before taking this medication, let your doctor know if you have active infection, liver or kidney disease or underlying cancer. Your doctor should order periodic tests to check for the drug's effect on the blood. Either member of a couple who is taking leflunomide and is ready to conceive should go through an elimination process using the drug cholestyramine prior to conception.

Leukeran

Generic name:
Chlorambucil

Type of medication: DMARD

What it's used for: Severe rheumatoid arthritis

Dosage: 2 to 8 mg per day in 1 or 2 doses

Special instructions: Use only for life-threatening organ disease.

Possible side effects: Hair loss, low blood counts, missing menstrual periods, nausea

Be aware: Before taking this drug, let your doctor know if you have active infection. Use of this drug may make you more susceptible to infections and certain cancers.

Lodine

Generic name:
Etodolac

Other brand name(s):
Lodine XL

Type of medication: NSAID

What it's used for: To ease arthritis pain and inflammation

Dosage: 600 to 1,200 mg per day in 2 or 4 doses

Special instructions: Do not take with other prescription or OTC NSAIDs. Take as directed at the same times every day. If you experience stomach upset, take with food, a glass of milk or an antacid.

Possible side effects: Abdominal or stomach cramps, pain or discomfort; diarrhea; dizziness; drowsiness; edema (swelling of feet); gastrointestinal bleeding; headache; heartburn or indigestion; nausea or vomiting; peptic ulcer

Be aware: Before taking this medication, let your doctor know if you drink alcohol or use blood thinners or if you have or have had any of the following: sensitivity or allergy to aspirin or similar drugs, kidney or liver disease, heart disease, high blood pressure, asthma or stomach ulcers. Because stomach ulcers or internal bleeding can occur without warning, regular checkups are important. Patients on long-term NSAIDs should have blood counts and liver enzymes checked periodically.

Unlike low-dose aspirin, there is little evidence that this or other NSAIDs will protect against heart attack or stroke. NSAIDs may be used with low-dose aspirin, but doing so may slightly increase your risk of gastric bleeding. Before taking this or any NSAID, tell your doctor if you take ACE inhibitors, lithium, warfarin or furosemide.

All NSAIDs may cause an increased risk of serious blood clots, heart attacks and stroke, which can be fatal. This risk may increase with dose and duration of use. Patients with cardiovascular disease or risk factors for cardiovascular disease may be at higher risk. These drugs should not be used for pain in people having coronary bypass surgery.

Lodine XL, see Etodolac

Lopurin

Generic name:
Allopurinol

Other brand name(s):
Zyloprim

Type of medication: Uric-acid-lowering drug

What it's used for: Gout

Dosage: 100 to 800 mg per day in a single dose. The dose is adjusted to achieve a serum uric acid level of lower than 6 mg/dl

Special instructions: Take immediately after a meal. Stop taking at the first sign of a rash, which may indicate an allergic reaction.

Possible side effects: Skin rash, hives or itching

Be aware: Before taking this drug, let your doctor know if you use azathioprine (*Imuran*) or if you have kidney disease. Acute gout attacks are common when this drug is started. These attacks can be minimized by taking lower doses and by taking the drug with colchicine or NSAIDs. Never start or stop this drug during a flare.

Lorcet

Generic name:
Hydrocodone with acetaminophen

Other brand name(s):
Dolacet, Hydrocet, Lortab, Vicodin

Type of medication: Analgesic

What it's used for: Pain not relieved by plain acetaminophen

Dosage: 2.5 to 10 mg every 4 to 6 hours as needed (Acetaminophen portion of medication varies)

Special instructions: Do not increase dose on your own because side effects increase and tolerance develops as dosage increases; do not stop abruptly unless advised to do so by your doctor; do not drive or operate heavy machinery until you know how your body reacts to this drug.

Possible side effects: Constipation, dizziness, lightheadedness, mood changes, nausea, sedation, shortness of breath, vomiting and urinary retention

Be aware: If you consume 3 or more alcoholic drinks per day, consult your doctor before taking acetaminophen. Mixing alcohol with acetaminophen can cause liver damage. Over time, this drug may cause psychological and physical dependence. Before taking this drug, let your doctor know if you use central nervous system depressants, such as antihistamines (allergy medications), tranquilizers, sleeping medications, muscle relaxants or narcotic pain medication, or if you have one of the following: liver disease, or history or alcohol or drug abuse.

Lortab

Generic name:
Hydrocodone with acetaminophen

Other brand name(s):
Dolacet, Hydrocet, Lorcet, Vicodin

Type of medication: Analgesic

What it's used for: Pain not relieved by plain acetaminophen

Dosage: 2.5 to 10 mg every 4 to 6 hours as needed (Acetaminophen portion of medication varies)

Special instructions: Do not increase dose on your own because side effects increase and tolerance develops as dosage increases; do not stop abruptly unless advised to do so by your doctor; do not drive or operate heavy machinery until you know how your body reacts to this drug.

Possible side effects: Constipation, dizziness, lightheadedness, mood changes, nausea, sedation, shortness of breath, vomiting and urinary retention

Be aware: If you consume 3 or more alcoholic drinks per day, consult your doctor before taking acetaminophen. Mixing alcohol with acetaminophen can cause liver damage. Over time, this drug may cause psychological and physical dependence. Before taking this drug, let your doctor know if you use central nervous system depressants, such as antihistamines (allergy medications), tranquilizers, sleeping medications, muscle relaxants or narcotic pain medication, or if you have one of the following: liver disease, or history or alcohol or drug abuse.

M-p

Magan, see Magnesium salicylate

Magnesium salicylate

Brand name(s):
Prescription: Magan, Mobidin, Mobogesic
Non-prescription: Arthritab, Bayer Select, Doan's Pills

Type of medication: NSAID (nonacetylated salicylate)

What it's used for: To ease arthritis pain and inflammation

Dosage: 2,600 to 4,800 mg per day in 3 to 6 doses

Special instructions: Take with food. Do not chew tablets. Do not crush enteric-coated or time-release forms and mix with water. Do not combine with other NSAIDs.

Possible side effects: Abdominal or stomach cramps; pain or discomfort; diarrhea; dizziness; drowsiness; edema (swelling of the feet); gastrointestinal bleeding; headache; heartburn or indigestion; nausea or vomiting; peptic ulcer

Be aware: Dizziness, deafness or ringing in the ears indicate that you are taking too much. Before taking these medications, let your doctor know if you drink alcohol or use other NSAIDs. If you are taking doses of more than 3,600 mg per day, your doctor should monitor salicylate levels in your blood.

Marthritic

Generic name:
Salsalate

Other brand name(s):
Amigesic, Anaflex 750, Disalcid, Mono-Gesic, Salflex, Salsitab

Type of medication: NSAID (nonacetylated salicylate)

What it's used for: To ease arthritis pain and inflammation

Dosage: 1,000 to 3,000 mg per day in 2 or 3 doses

Special instructions: Take with food. Do not chew tablets. Do not crush enteric-coated or time-release forms and mix with water. Do not combine with other NSAIDs.

Possible side effects: Abdominal or stomach cramps, pain or discomfort; diarrhea; dizziness; drowsiness; edema (swelling of the feet); gastrointestinal bleeding; headache; heartburn or indigestion; nausea or vomiting; peptic ulcer

Be aware: Dizziness, deafness or ringing in the ears indicate that you are taking too much. Before taking these medications, let your doctor know if you drink alcohol or use other NSAIDs. If you are taking doses of more than 3,600 mg per day, your doctor should monitor salicylate levels in your blood.

Meclofenamate sodium

Brand name(s):
Meclomen

Type of medication: NSAID

What it's used for: To ease arthritis pain and inflammation

Dosage: 200 to 400 mg per day in 4 doses

Special instructions: Do not take with other prescription or OTC NSAIDs. Take as directed at the same time(s) every day. If you experience stomach upset, take with food, a glass of milk or an antacid.

Possible side effects: Abdominal or stomach cramps, pain or discomfort; diarrhea; dizziness; edema (swelling of the feet); headache; gastrointestinal bleeding; heartburn or indigestion; nausea or vomiting; peptic ulcer

Be aware: Before taking this medication, let your doctor know if you drink alcohol or use blood thinners, or if you have or have had any of the following: sensitivity or allergy to aspirin or similar drugs, kidney or liver disease, heart disease, high blood pressure, asthma or stomach ulcers. Because stomach ulcers or internal bleeding can occur without warning, regular checkups are important. Patients on long-term NSAIDs should have blood counts and liver enzymes checked periodically.

Unlike low-dose aspirin, there is little evidence that this or other NSAIDs will protect against heart attack or stroke.

NSAIDs may be used with low-dose aspirin, but doing so may slightly increase your risk of gastric bleeding. Before taking this or any NSAID, tell your doctor if you take ACE inhibitors, lithium, warfarin or furosemide.

All NSAIDs may cause an increased risk of serious blood clots, heart attacks and stroke, which can be fatal. This risk may increase with dose and duration of use. Patients with cardiovascular disease or risk factors for cardiovascular disease may be at higher risk. These drugs should not be used for pain in people having coronary bypass surgery.

Meclomen, see Meclofenamate sodium

Medrol

Generic name:
Methylprednisolone

Type of medication: Corticosteroid

What it's used for: To control inflammation of joints and organs in many forms of arthritis and related conditions

Dosage: Dosage varies widely according to the disease being treated. Taking either too much or too little can be dangerous. Take exactly the amount prescribed by your doctor.

Special instructions: Take with food. A single daily dose should be taken with breakfast. Sometimes the dose is split, taken 2 to 4 times a day. Don't stop medication abruptly; dosage must be tapered or reduced gradually.

Possible side effects: Bruising, cataracts, elevated blood fats (triglycerides, cholesterol), elevated blood sugar, hardening of the arteries (atherosclerosis), hypertension, increased appetite, indigestion, insomnia, mood swings, muscle weakness, nervousness or restlessness, osteoporosis, susceptibility to infection, thin skin

Be aware: Before taking this medication, let your doctor know if you have one of the following: fungal infection, history of tuberculosis, underactive thyroid, diabetes, stomach ulcer, high blood pressure or osteoporosis. If you are allergic to FD&C, No. 5, do not take the 24-mg tablet of *Medrol*.

Mefenamic acid

Brand name(s):
Ponstel

Type of medication: NSAID

What it's used for: To ease arthritis pain and inflammation

Dosage: 500 mg initial dose, 250 mg every 6 hours as needed, for up to 7 days

Special instructions: Do not take with other prescription or OTC NSAIDs. Take as directed at the same time(s) every day. If you experience stomach upset, take with food, a glass of milk or antacid.

Possible side effects: Abdominal or stomach cramps, pain or discomfort; diarrhea; dizziness; edema (swelling of the feet); headache; gastrointestinal bleeding; heartburn or indigestion; nausea or vomiting; peptic ulcer

Be aware: Before taking this medication, let your doctor know if you drink alcohol or use blood thinners or if you have or have had any of the following: sensitivity or allergy to aspirin or similar drugs, kidney or liver disease, heart disease, high blood pressure, asthma or stomach ulcers. Because stomach ulcers or internal bleeding can occur without warning, regular checkups are important.

Unlike low-dose aspirin, there is little evidence that this or other NSAIDs will protect against heart attack or stroke. NSAIDs may be used with low-dose aspirin, but doing so may slightly increase your risk of gastric bleeding. Before taking this or any NSAID, tell your doctor if you take ACE inhibitors, lithium, warfarin or furosemide.

This medication is for short-term relief of pain and should not be used for more than 7 days.

All NSAIDs may cause an increased risk of serious blood clots, heart attacks and stroke, which can be fatal. This risk may increase with dose and duration of use. Patients with cardiovascular disease or risk factors for cardiovascular disease may be at higher risk. These drugs should not be used for pain in people having coronary bypass surgery.

Meloxicam

Brand name(s):
Mobic

Type of medication: NSAID

What it's used for: To ease arthritis pain and inflammation

Dosage: 7.5 to 15 mg per day in a single dose

Special instructions: Do not take with other prescription or OTC NSAIDs. Take as directed at the same time(s) every day. If you experience stomach upset, take with food, a glass of milk or an antacid.

Possible side effects: Abdominal or stomach cramps, pain or discomfort; diarrhea; dizziness; edema (swelling of the feet); headache; gastrointestinal bleeding; heartburn or indigestion; nausea or vomiting; peptic ulcer

Be aware: Before taking this medication, let your doctor know if you drink alcohol or use blood thinners, or if you have or have had any of the following: sensitivity or allergy to aspirin or similar drugs, kidney or liver disease, heart disease, high blood pressure, asthma or stomach ulcers. Because stomach ulcers or internal bleeding can occur without warning, regular checkups are important. Patients on long-term NSAIDs should have blood counts and liver enzymes checked periodically.

Unlike low-dose aspirin, there is little evidence that this or other NSAIDs will protect against heart attack or stroke.

NSAIDs may be used with low-dose aspirin, but doing so may slightly increase your risk of gastric bleeding. Before taking this or any NSAID, tell your doctor if you tale ACE inhibitors, lithium, warfarin or furosemide.

All NSAIDs may cause an increased risk of serious blood clots, heart attacks and stroke, which can be fatal. This risk may increase with dose and duration of use. Patients with cardiovascular disease or risk factors for cardiovascular disease may be at higher risk. These drugs should not be used for pain in pcople having coronary bypass surgery.

Menest, see Estrogens

Menostar, see Estrogens

Methotrexate

Brand name(s):
Rheumatrex, Trexall

Type of medication: DMARD

What it's used for: Rheumatoid arthritis, lupus, and other forms of arthritis

Dosage: 7.5 to 20 mg per week in a single dose orally (this drug may also be given by injection)

Possible side effects: Abdominal discomfort, chills, dizziness, fever, general feeling of illness, hair loss, headache, increased sun sensitivity, itching, liver problems, low blood counts, mouth sores, nausea and stomach upset, rashes, shortness of breath, sleepiness, weakness

Be aware: Let your doctor know if you have one of the following: abnormal blood count, liver or lung disease, alcoholism, active infection or hepatitis. Your doctor should order chest X-rays, liver tests and blood counts before you start this drug and throughout treatment to monitor for side effects. Alert your doctor immediately if you have a dry cough, fever or difficulty breathing. This drug can rarely be associated with increased risk of blood diseases such as lymphoma.

Methylprednisolone

Brand name(s):
Medrol

Type of medication: Corticosteroid

What it's used for: To control inflammation of joints and organs in many forms of arthritis and related conditions

Dosage: Dosage varies widely according to the disease being treated. Taking either too much or too little can be dangerous. Take exactly the amount prescribed by your doctor.

Special instructions: Take with food. A single daily dose should be taken with breakfast. Sometimes the dose is split, taken 2 to 4 times a day. Don't stop medication abruptly; dosage must be tapered or reduced gradually.

Possible side effects: Bruising, cataracts, elevated blood fats (triglycerides, cholesterol), elevated blood sugar, hardening of the arteries (atherosclerosis), hypertension, increased appetite, indigestion, insomnia, mood swings, muscle weakness, nervousness or restlessness, osteoporosis, susceptibility to infection, thin skin

Be aware: Before taking this medication, let your doctor know if you have one of the following: fungal infection, history of tuberculosis, underactive thyroid, diabetes, stomach ulcer, high blood pressure or osteoporosis. If you are allergic to FD&C, No. 5, do not take the 24-mg tablet of *Medrol.*

Miacalcin

Generic name:
Calcitonin (nasal spray)

Type of medication: Parathyroid hormone

What it's used for: Osteoporosis

Dosage: 200 IUs per day in a single dose

Special instructions: Alternate nostrils daily. Store medication in refrigerator prior to opening. Store at room temperature after opening.

Possible side effects: Crusting, patches or sores inside the nose; dryness, itching, redness, swelling, tenderness or other signs of nasal irritation; nosebleeds; runny nose

Be aware: Before taking this drug, let your doctor know if you have a protein allergy.

Minocin, see Minocycline

Minocycline

Brand name(s):
Minocin

Type of medication: Antibiotic, DMARD

What it's used for: Rheumatoid arthritis, osteoarthritis

Dosage: 200 mg per day in 2 or 4 doses

Special instructions: Take on an empty stomach. Swallow whole with water. Drink plenty of fluids.

Possible side effects: Cramps or burning of the stomach; diarrhea; darkening of the skin; dizziness, lightheadedness or unsteadiness; liver problems; sun sensitivity

Be aware: This drug is not currently FDA approved for arthritis. It is an antibiotic. Before taking this medication, let your doctor know if you have a sensitivity to tetracycline products. In children, minocycline can cause permanent tooth discoloration.

Mobic

Generic name:
Meloxicam

Type of medication: NSAID

What it's used for: To ease arthritis pain and inflammation

Dosage: 7.5 to 15 mg per day in a single dose

Special instructions: Do not take with other prescription or OTC NSAIDs. Take as directed at the same time(s) every day. If you experience stomach upset, take with food, a glass of milk or an antacid.

Possible side effects: Abdominal or stomach cramps, pain or discomfort; diarrhea; dizziness; edema (swelling of the feet); gastrointestinal bleeding; headache; heartburn or indigestion; nausea or vomiting; peptic ulcer

Be aware: Before taking this medication, let your doctor know if you drink alcohol or use blood thinners, or if you have or have had any of the following: sensitivity or allergy to aspirin or similar drugs, kidney or liver disease, heart disease, high blood pressure, asthma or stomach ulcers. Because stomach ulcers or internal bleeding can occur without warning, regular checkups are important. Patients on long-term NSAIDs should have blood counts and liver enzymes checked periodically.

Unlike low-dose aspirin, there is little evidence that this or other NSAIDs will protect against heart attack or stroke. NSAIDs may be used with low-dose aspirin, but doing so may slightly increase your risk of gastric bleeding. Before taking this or any NSAID, tell your doctor if you tale ACE inhibitors, lithium, warfarin or furosemide.

All NSAIDs may cause an increased risk of serious blood clots, heart attacks and stroke, which can be fatal. This risk may increase with dose and duration of use. Patients with cardiovascular disease or risk factors for cardiovascular disease may be at higher risk. These drugs should not be used for pain in people having coronary bypass surgery.

Mobidin

Generic name:
Magnesium salicylate

Other brand name(s):
Prescription: Magan, Mobogesic
Non-prescription: Arthritab, Bayer Select, Doan's Pills

Type of medication: NSAID (nonacetylated salicylate)

What it's used for: To ease arthritis pain and inflammation

Dosage: 2,600 to 4,800 mg per day in 3 to 6 doses

Special instructions: Take with food. Do not chew tablets. Do not crush enteric-coated or time-release forms and mix with water. Do not combine with other NSAIDs.

Possible side effects: Abdominal or stomach cramps; pain or discomfort; diarrhea; dizziness; drowsiness; edema (swelling of the feet); gastrointestinal bleeding; headache; heartburn or indigestion; nausea or vomiting; peptic ulcer

Be aware: Dizziness, deafness or ringing in the ears indicates that you are taking too much. Before taking these medications, let your doctor know if you drink alcohol or use other NSAIDs. If you are taking doses of more than 3,600 mg per day, your doctor should monitor salicylate levels in your blood.

Mobogesic

Generic name:
Magnesium salicylate

Other brand name(s):
Prescription: Magan, Mobidin
Non-prescription: Arthritab, Bayer Select, Doan's Pills

Type of medication: NSAID (nonacetylated salicylate)

What it's used for: To ease arthritis pain and inflammation

Dosage: 2,600 to 4,800 mg per day in 3 to 6 doses

Special instructions: Take with food. Do not chew tablets. Do not crush enteric-coated or time-release forms and mix with water. Do not combine with other NSAIDs.

Possible side effects: Abdominal or stomach cramps, pain or discomfort; diarrhea; dizziness; drowsiness; edema (swelling of the feet); gastrointestinal bleeding; headache; heartburn or indigestion; nausea or vomiting; peptic ulcer

Be aware: Dizziness, deafness or ringing in the ears indicates that you are taking too much. Before taking these medications, let your doctor know if you drink alcohol or use other NSAIDs. If you are taking doses of more than 3,600 mg per day, your doctor should monitor salicylate levels in your blood.

Mono-Gesic

Generic name:
Salsalate

Other brand name(s):
Amigesic, Anaflex 750, Disalcid, Marthritic, Salflex, Salsitab

Type of medication: NSAID (nonacetylated salicylate)

What it's used for: To ease arthritis pain and inflammation

Dosage: 1,000 to 3,000 mg per day in 2 or 3 doses

Special instructions: Take with food. Do not chew tablets. Do not crush enteric-coated or time-release forms and mix with water. Do not combine with other NSAIDs.

Possible side effects: Abdominal or stomach cramps, pain or discomfort; diarrhea; dizziness; drowsiness; edema (swelling of the feet); gastrointestinal bleeding; headache; heartburn or indigestion; nausea or vomiting; peptic ulcer

Be aware: Dizziness, deafness or ringing in the ears indicates that you are taking too much. Before taking these medications, let your doctor know if you drink alcohol or use other NSAIDs. If you are taking doses of more than 3,600 mg per day, your doctor should monitor salicylate levels in your blood.

Morphine sulfate

Brand name(s):
Avinza, Oramorph SR

Type of medication: Analgesic (narcotic)

What it's used for: To ease severe pain associated with arthritis, surgery and fractures

Dosage: 30 mg per day in a single dose to start. Doctor may increase dose as necessary (*Avinza*); 30 to 100 mg every 12 hours as needed (*Oramorph SR*)

Special instructions: Take at the same times each day with or without food. Swallow whole. Do not chew or crush. Do not stop drug abruptly. Do not drive or use heavy machinery until you know how your body reacts to this drug.

Possible side effects: Constipation, drowsiness, nausea

Be aware: Over time, this drug may cause psychological and physical dependence. Before taking this drug, let your doctor know if you use a central nervous system depressant, such antihistamines (allergy medications), tranquilizers, sleeping medications, muscle relaxants or narcotic pain medication, or if you have one of the following: liver disease, or history of alcohol or drug abuse.

Motrin

Generic name:
Ibuprofen

Other brand name(s):
Non-prescription: Advil, Motrin IB, Nuprin

Type of medication: NSAID

What it's used for: To ease arthritis pain and inflammation

Dosage: 1,200 to 3,200 mg per day in 3 or 4 doses

Special instructions: Do not take for more than 10 days for pain or more than three days for fever unless directed by a doctor. Do not take with other prescription or OTC NSAIDs. Take as directed at the same time(s) every day. If stomach upset occurs, take with food, a glass of milk or an antacid.

Possible side effects: Abdominal or stomach cramps, pain or discomfort; diarrhea; dizziness; edema (swelling of the feet); gastrointestinal bleeding; headache; heartburn or indigestion; nausea or vomiting; peptic ulcer

Be aware: Before taking this medication, let your doctor know if you drink alcohol or use blood thinners, or if you have or have had any of the following: sensitivity or allergy to aspirin or similar drugs, kidney or liver disease, heart disease, high blood pressure, asthma or stomach ulcers. Because stomach ulcers or internal bleeding can occur without warning, regular checkups are important. Patients on long-term NSAIDs should have blood counts and liver enzymes checked periodically.

Unlike low-dose aspirin, there is little evidence that this drug or other NSAIDs will protect against heart attack or stroke. NSAIDs may be used with low-dose aspirin, but doing so may slightly increase your risk of gastric bleeding. Before taking this or any NSAID, tell your doctor if you take ACE inhibitors, lithium, warfarin or furosemide.

All NSAIDs may cause an increased risk of serious blood clots, heart attacks and stroke, which can be fatal. This risk may increase with dose and duration of use. Patients with cardiovascular disease or risk factors for cardiovascular disease may be at higher risk. These drugs should not be used for pain in people having coronary bypass surgery.

Motrin IB

Generic name:
Ibuprofen

Other brand name(s):
Prescription: Motrin
Non-prescription: Advil, Nuprin

Type of medication: NSAID

What it's used for: To ease arthritis pain and inflammation

Dosage: 200 to 400 mg every 4 to 6 hours as needed; no more than 1,200 mg per day

Special instructions: Do not take for more than 10 days for pain or more than three days for fever unless directed by a doctor. Do not take with other prescription or OTC NSAIDs. Take as directed at the same time(s) every day. If stomach upset occurs, take with food, a glass of milk or an antacid.

Possible side effects: Abdominal or stomach cramps, pain or discomfort; diarrhea; dizziness; edema (swelling of the feet); gastrointestinal bleeding; headache; heartburn or indigestion; nausea or vomiting; peptic ulcer

Be aware: Before taking this medication, let your doctor know if you drink alcohol or use blood thinners, or if you have or have had any of the following: sensitivity or allergy to aspirin or similar drugs, kidney or liver disease, heart disease, high blood pressure, asthma or stomach ulcers. Because stomach ulcers or internal bleeding can occur

without warning, regular checkups are important. Patients on long-term NSAIDs should have blood counts and liver enzymes checked periodically.

Unlike low-dose aspirin, there is little evidence that this drug or other NSAIDs will protect against heart attack or stroke. NSAIDs may be used with low-dose aspirin, but doing so may slightly increase your risk of gastric bleeding. Before taking this or any NSAID, tell your doctor if you take ACE inhibitors, lithium, warfarin or furosemide.

All NSAIDs may cause an increased risk of serious blood clots, heart attacks and stroke, which can be fatal. This risk may increase with dose and duration of use. Patients with cardiovascular disease or risk factors for cardiovascular disease may be at higher risk. These drugs should not be used for pain in people having coronary bypass surgery.

Myochrysine

Generic name:
Gold sodium thiomalate (injectable gold)

Type of medication: DMARD

What it's used for: Rheumatoid arthritis

Dosage: 10 mg in a single injection the first week, 25 mg the following week, then 25 to 50 mg per week thereafter. Frequency may be reduced after several months.

Possible side effects: Irritation and soreness of tongue; irritated or bleeding of gums; metallic taste; skin rash or itching; ulcers, sores or white spots on lips or in mouth or throat

Be aware: Before taking this medication, let your doctor know if you have any of the following: lupus, skin rash, kidney disease or colitis. Increased joint pain may occur for 1 or 2 days after injection, but it usually disappears after the first few injections. Your doctor should order periodic urine and blood tests to check for side effects.

Nabumetone

Brand name(s):
Relafen

Type of medication: NSAID

What it's used for: To ease arthritis pain and inflammation

Dosage: 1,000 mg per day in 1 or 2 doses; 2,000 mg per day in 2 doses

Special instructions: Do not take with other prescription or OTC NSAIDs. Take as directed at the same time(s) every day. If you experience stomach upset, take with food, a glass of milk or an antacid.

Possible side effects: Abdominal or stomach cramps, pain or discomfort; diarrhea; dizziness; edema (swelling of the feet); gastrointestinal bleeding; headache; heartburn or indigestion; nausea or vomiting; peptic ulcer

Be aware: Before taking this medication, let your doctor know if you drink alcohol or use blood thinners, or if you have or have had any of the following: sensitivity or allergy to aspirin or similar drugs, kidney or liver disease, heart disease, high blood pressure, asthma or stomach ulcers. Because stomach ulcers or internal bleeding can occur without warning, regular checkups are important. Patients on long-term NSAIDs should have blood counts and liver enzymes checked periodically.

Unlike low-dose aspirin, there is little evidence that this or other NSAIDs will protect against heart attack or stroke. NSAIDs may be used with low dose aspirin, but doing so may slightly increase your risk of gastric bleeding. Before taking this or any NSAID, tell your doctor if you take ACE inhibitors, lithium, warfarin or furosemide.

All NSAIDs may cause an increased risk of serious blood clots, heart attacks and stroke, which can be fatal. This risk may increase with dose and duration of use. Patients with cardiovascular disease or risk factors for cardiovascular disease may be at higher risk. These drugs should not be used for pain in people having coronary bypass surgery.

Nalfon

Generic name:
Fenoprofen calcium

Type of medication: NSAID

What it's used for: To ease arthritis pain and inflammation

Dosage: 900 to 2,400 mg per day in 3 or 4 doses; never more than 3,200 mg per day

Special instructions: Do not take with other prescription or OTC NSAIDs. Take as directed at the same time(s) every day. If you experience stomach upset, take with food, a glass of milk or an antacid.

Possible side effects: Abdominal or stomach cramps, pain or discomfort; diarrhea; dizziness; edema (swelling of the feet); headache; gastrointestinal bleeding; heartburn or indigestion; nausea or vomiting; peptic ulcer

Be aware: Before taking this medication, let your doctor know if you drink alcohol or use blood thinners or if you have or have had any of the following: sensitivity or allergy to aspirin or similar drugs, kidney or liver disease, heart disease, high blood pressure, asthma or stomach ulcers. Because stomach ulcers or internal bleeding can occur without warning, regular checkups are important. Patients on long-term NSAIDs should have blood counts and liver enzymes checked periodically.

Unlike low-dose aspirin, there is little evidence that this or other NSAIDs will protect against heart attack or stroke. NSAIDs may be used with low-dose aspirin, but doing so may slightly increase your risk of gastric bleeding. Before taking this or any NSAID, tell your doctor if you take ACE inhibitors, lithium, warfarin or furosemide.

All NSAIDs may cause an increased risk of serious blood clots, heart attacks and stroke, which can be fatal. This risk may increase with dose and duration of use. Patients with cardiovascular disease or risk factors for cardiovascular disease may be at higher risk. These drugs should not be used for pain in people having coronary bypass surgery.

Naprelan, see naproxen

Naprosyn, see naproxen

Naproxen

Brand name(s):
Naprosyn, Naprelan

Type of medication: NSAID

What it's used for: To ease arthritis pain and inflammation

Dosage: 500 to 1,500 mg per day in 2 doses (*Naprosyn*); 750 to 1,000 mg per day in a single dose (*Naprelan*)

Special instructions: Do not take with other prescription or OTC NSAIDs. Take as directed at the same time(s) every day. If you experience stomach upset, take with food, a glass of milk or an antacid.

Possible side effects: Abdominal or stomach cramps, pain or discomfort; diarrhea; dizziness; edema (swelling of the feet); headache; gastrointestinal bleeding; heartburn or indigestion; nausea or vomiting; peptic ulcer

Be aware: Before taking this medication, let your doctor know if you drink alcohol or use blood thinners or if you have or have had any of the following: sensitivity or allergy to aspirin or similar drugs, kidney or liver disease, heart disease, high blood pressure, asthma or stomach ulcers. Because stomach ulcers or internal bleeding can occur without warning, regular checkups are important. Patients on long-term NSAIDs should have blood counts and liver enzymes checked periodically.

Unlike low-dose aspirin, there is little evidence that this or other NSAIDs will protect against heart attack or stroke. NSAIDs may be used with low-dose aspirin, but doing so may slightly increase your risk of gastric bleeding. Before taking this or any NSAID, tell your doctor if you take ACE inhibitors, lithium, warfarin or furosemide.

All NSAIDs may cause an increased risk of serious blood clots, heart attacks and stroke, which can be fatal. This risk may increase with dose and duration of use. Patients with cardiovascular disease or risk factors for cardiovascular disease may be at higher risk. These drugs should not be used for pain in people having coronary bypass surgery.

Naproxen sodium

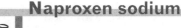

Brand name(s):
Prescription: Anaprox
Non-prescription: Aleve

Type of medication: NSAID

What it's used for: To ease arthritis pain and inflammation

Dosage: 550 to 1,650 mg per day in 2 doses (prescription); 220 mg every 8 to 12 hours as needed (non-prescription)

Special instructions: Do not take with other prescription or OTC NSAIDs. Take as directed at the same time(s) every day. If you experience stomach upset, take with food, a glass of milk or an antacid.

Possible side effects: Abdominal or stomach cramps, pain or discomfort; diarrhea; dizziness; edema (swelling of the feet); headache; gastrointestinal bleeding; heartburn or indigestion; nausea or vomiting; peptic ulcer

Be aware: Before taking this medication, let your doctor know if you drink alcohol or use blood thinners or if you have or have had any of the following: sensitivity or allergy to aspirin or similar drugs, kidney or liver disease, heart disease, high blood pressure, asthma or stomach ulcers. Because stomach ulcers or internal bleeding can occur without warning, regular checkups are important. Patients on long-term NSAIDs should have blood counts and liver enzymes checked periodically.

Unlike low-dose aspirin, there is little evidence that this or other NSAIDs will protect against heart attack or stroke. NSAIDs may be used with low-dose aspirin, but doing so may slightly increase your risk of gastric bleeding. Before taking this or any NSAID, tell your doctor if you take ACE inhibitors, lithium, warfarin or furosemide.

All NSAIDs may cause an increased risk of serious blood clots, heart attacks and stroke, which can be fatal. This risk may increase with dose and duration of use. Patients with cardiovascular disease or risk factors for cardiovascular disease may be at higher risk. These drugs should not be used for pain in people having coronary bypass surgery.

Neoral

Generic name:
Cyclosporine

Type of medication: DMARD

What it's used for: To slow the progression of rheumatoid arthritis

Dosage: 100 to 400 mg per day in 2 doses. Exact doses vary by patient weight.

Special instructions: Take at the same times every day, either with meals or between meals.

Possible side effects: Headache, high blood pressure, increase in hair growth, kidney problems, loss of appetite, nausea

Be aware: Before taking this drug, tell your doctor if you have liver or kidney disease, active infection or high blood pressure. Because this drug's rate of absorption is unpredictable, your doctor should monitor it through blood tests. Use of this drug may make you more susceptible to infection and certain cancers. Do not take with St. John's wort, grapefruit or grapefruit juice.

Nuprin

Generic name:
Ibuprofen

Other brand name(s):
Prescription: Motrin
Non-prescription: Advil, Motrin IB

Type of medication: NSAID (OTC)

What it's used for: To ease arthritis pain and inflammation

Dosage: 200 to 400 mg every 4 to 6 hours as needed, no more than 1,200 mg per day (non-prescription)

Special instructions: Do not take for more than 10 days for pain or more than three days for fever unless directed by a doctor. Do not take with other prescription or OTC NSAIDs. Take as directed at the same time(s) every day. If stomach upset occurs, take with food, a glass of milk or an antacid.

Possible side effects: Abdominal or stomach cramps, pain or discomfort; diarrhea; dizziness; edema (swelling of the feet); headache; gastrointestinal bleeding; heartburn or indigestion; nausea or vomiting; peptic ulcer

Be aware: Before taking this medication, let your doctor know if you drink alcohol or use blood thinners, or if you have or have had any of the following: sensitivity or allergy to aspirin or similar drugs, kidney or liver disease, heart disease, high blood pressure, asthma or stomach ulcers. Because stomach ulcers or internal bleeding can occur without warning, regular checkups are important. Patients on long-term NSAIDs should have blood counts and liver enzymes checked periodically.

Unlike low-dose aspirin, there is little evidence that this drug or other NSAIDs will protect against heart attack or stroke. NSAIDs may be used with low-dose aspirin, but doing so may slightly increase your risk of gastric bleeding. Before taking this or any NSAID, tell your doctor if you take ACE inhibitors, lithium, warfarin or furosemide.

All NSAIDs may cause an increased risk of serious blood clots, heart attacks and stroke, which can be fatal. This risk may increase with dose and duration of use. Patients with cardiovascular disease or risk factors for cardiovascular disease may be at higher risk. These drugs should not be used for pain in people having coronary bypass surgery.

Oramorph SR

Generic name:
Morphine sulfate

Other brand name(s):
Avinza

Type of medication: Analgesic

What it's used for: To ease severe pain associated with arthritis, surgery and fractures

Dosage: 30 to 100 mg every 12 hours as needed

Special instructions: Take at the same times each day with or without food. Swallow whole. Do not chew or crush. Do not stop drug abruptly. Do not drive or use heavy machinery until you know how your body reacts to this drug.

Possible side effects: Constipation, drowsiness, nausea

Be aware: Over time, this drug may cause psychological and physical dependence. Before taking this drug, let your doctor know if you use a central nervous system depressant, such antihistamines (allergy medications), tranquilizers, sleeping medications, muscle relaxants or narcotic pain medication, or if you have one of the following: liver disease, or history of alcohol or drug abuse.

Orasone

Generic name:
Prednisone

Other brand name(s):
Deltasone, Prednicen-M, Sterapred

Type of medication: Corticosteroid

What it's used for: To control inflammation of joints and organs in many forms of arthritis and related conditions

Dosage: Dosage varies widely according to the disease being treated. Taking either too much or too little can be dangerous. Take exactly the amount prescribed by your doctor.

Special instructions: Take with food. A single daily dose should be taken with breakfast. Sometimes the dose is split, taken 2 to 4 times per day. Don't stop medication abruptly; dosage must be tapered or reduced gradually.

Possible side effects: Bruising, cataracts, elevated blood fats (cholesterol, triglycerides), elevated blood sugar, hardening of the arteries (atherosclerosis), hypertension, increased appetite, indigestion, insomnia, mood swings, muscle weakness, nervousness or restlessness, osteoporosis, susceptibility to infection, thin skin

Be aware: Before taking this medication, let your doctor know if you have one of the following: fungal infection, history of tuberculosis, underactive thyroid, diabetes, stomach ulcer, high blood pressure or osteoporosis.

Orencia

Generic name:
abatacept

Type of medication: Biologic response modifier

What it's used for: Moderate to severe rheumatoid arthritis

Dosage: Dose is based on body weight and ranges from 500 mg to 1 gram for most people. After three initial infusions at 0, 2 and 4 weeks, infusions are repeated every 4 weeks.

Special instructions: Drug is given intravenously through a vein in the arm during a 30-minute infusion done in a doctor's office, clinic or hospital. *Orencia* can be given along with disease-modifying antirheumatic drugs.

Possible side effects: Cough; dizziness; headache; infusion reactions, including change in blood pressure, facial swelling, hives, trouble breathing; serious infections; sore throat

Be aware: Rheumatoid arthritis carries a higher risk of infection and lymphoma. It is uncertain whether this and other biologic response modifiers increase lymphoma risk. This agent should be discontinued if you have a serious or recurrent infection, exposure to tuberculosis or positive skin test for tuberculosis. *Orencia* should be used with caution in patients with congestive heart failure (CHF).

Orudis

Generic name:
Ketoprofen

Other brand name(s):
Prescription: Oruvail
Non-prescription: Actron, Orudis KT

Type of medication: NSAID

What it's used for: To ease arthritis pain and inflammation

Dosage: 200 to 225 mg per day in 3 or 4 doses

Special instructions: Do not take with other prescription or OTC NSAIDs. Take as directed at the same times every day. If you experience stomach upset, take with food, a glass of milk or an antacid.

Possible side effects: Abdominal or stomach cramps, pain or discomfort; diarrhea; dizziness; edema (swelling of the feet); headache; gastrointestinal bleeding; heartburn or indigestion; nausea or vomiting; peptic ulcer

Be aware: Before taking this medication, let your doctor know if you drink alcohol or use blood thinners, or if you have or have had any of the following: sensitivity or allergy to aspirin or similar drugs, kidney or liver disease, heart disease, high blood pressure, asthma or stomach ulcers. Because stomach ulcers or internal bleeding can occur without warning, regular checkups are important. Patients on long-term NSAIDs should have blood counts and liver enzymes checked periodically.

Unlike low-dose aspirin, there is little evidence that this or other NSAIDs will protect against heart attack or stroke. NSAIDs may be used with low-dose aspirin, but doing so may slightly increase your risk of gastric bleeding. Before taking this or any NSAID, tell your doctor if you take ACE inhibitors, lithium, warfarin or furosemide.

All NSAIDs may cause an increased risk of serious blood clots, heart attacks and stroke, which can be fatal. This risk may increase with dose and duration of use. Patients with cardiovascular disease or risk factors for cardiovascular disease may be at higher risk. These drugs should not be used for pain in people having coronary bypass surgery.

Orudis KT

Generic name:
Ketoprofen

Other brand name(s):
Prescription: Orudis, Oruvail
Non-prescription: Actron

Type of medication: NSAID (OTC)

What it's used for: To ease arthritis pain and inflammation

Dosage: 12.5 mg every 4 to 6 hours as needed

Special instructions: Do not take for more than 10 days for pain or more than three days for fever unless directed by a doctor. Do not take with other prescription or OTC NSAIDs. Take as directed at the same time(s) every day. If you experience stomach upset, take with food or a glass of milk or an antacid.

Possible side effects: Abdominal or stomach cramps, pain or discomfort; diarrhea; dizziness; edema (swelling of the feet); headache; gastrointestinal bleeding; heartburn or indigestion; nausea or vomiting; peptic ulcer

Be aware: Before taking this medication, let your doctor know if you drink alcohol or use blood thinners, or if you have or have had any of the following: sensitivity or allergy to aspirin or similar drugs, kidney or liver disease, heart disease, high blood pressure, asthma or stomach ulcers. Because stomach ulcers or internal bleeding can occur without warning, regular checkups are important. Patients on long-term NSAIDs should have blood counts and liver enzymes checked periodically.

Unlike low-dose aspirin, there is little evidence that this or other NSAIDs will protect against heart attack or stroke. NSAIDs may be used with low-dose aspirin, but doing so may slightly increase your risk of gastric bleeding. Before taking this or any NSAID, tell your doctor if you take ACE inhibitors, lithium, warfarin or furosemide.

All NSAIDs may cause an increased risk of serious blood clots, heart attacks and stroke, which can be fatal. This risk may increase with dose and duration of use. Patients with cardiovascular disease or risk factors for cardiovascular disease may be at higher risk. These drugs should not be used for pain in people having coronary bypass surgery.

Oruvail

Generic name:
Ketoprofen

Other brand name(s):
Prescription: Orudis
Non-prescription: Actron, Orudis KT

Type of medication: NSAID

What it's used for: To ease arthritis pain and inflammation

Dosage: 150 or 200 mg per day in a single dose

Special instructions: Do not take with other prescription or OTC NSAIDs. Take as directed at the same times every day. If you experience stomach upset, take with food, a glass of milk or an antacid.

Possible side effects: Abdominal or stomach cramps, pain or discomfort; diarrhea; dizziness; edema (swelling of the feet); gastrointestinal bleeding; headache; heartburn or indigestion; nausea or vomiting; peptic ulcer

Be aware: Before taking this medication, let your doctor know if you drink alcohol or use blood thinners, or if you have or have had any of the following: sensitivity or allergy to aspirin or similar drugs, kidney or liver disease, heart disease, high blood pressure, asthma or stomach ulcers. Because stomach ulcers or internal bleeding can occur without warning, regular checkups are important. Patients on long-term NSAIDs should have blood counts and liver enzymes checked periodically.

Unlike low-dose aspirin, there is little evidence that this or other NSAIDs will protect against heart attack or stroke. NSAIDs may be used with low-dose aspirin, but doing so may slightly increase your risk of gastric bleeding. Before taking this or any NSAID, tell your doctor if you take ACE inhibitors, lithium, warfarin or furosemide.

All NSAIDs may cause an increased risk of serious blood clots, heart attacks and stroke, which can be fatal. This risk may increase with dose and duration of use. Patients with cardiovascular disease or risk factors for cardiovascular disease may be at higher risk. These drugs should not be used for pain in people having coronary bypass surgery.

Oxaprozin

Brand name(s):
Daypro

Type of medication: NSAID

What it's used for: To ease arthritis pain and inflammation

Dosage: 1,200 or 1,800 mg per day in a single dose

Special instructions: Do not take with other prescription or OTC NSAIDs. Take as directed at the same time every day. If you experience stomach upset, take with food, a glass of milk or an antacid.

Possible side effects: Abdominal or stomach cramps, pain or discomfort; diarrhea; dizziness; edema (swelling of the feet); headache; gastrointestinal bleeding; heartburn or indigestion; nausea or vomiting; peptic ulcer

Be aware: Before taking this medication, let your doctor know if you drink alcohol or use blood thinners or if you have or have had any of the following: sensitivity or allergy to aspirin or similar drugs, kidney or liver disease, heart disease, high blood pressure, asthma or stomach ulcers. Because stomach ulcers or internal bleeding can occur without warning, regular checkups are important. Patients on long-term NSAIDs should have blood counts and liver enzymes checked periodically.

Unlike low-dose aspirin, there is little evidence that this or other NSAIDs will protect against heart attack or stroke. NSAIDs may be used with low-dose aspirin, but doing so may slightly increase your risk of gastric bleeding. Before taking this or any NSAID, tell your doctor if you take ACE inhibitors, lithium, warfarin or furosemide.

All NSAIDs may cause an increased risk of serious blood clots, heart attacks and stroke, which can be fatal. This risk may increase with dose and duration of use. Patients with cardiovascular disease or risk factors for cardiovascular disease may be at higher risk. These drugs should not be used for pain in people having coronary bypass surgery.

Oxycodone

Brand name(s):
OxyContin, Roxicodone, OxyFAST, OxyIR (liquid)

Type of medication: Analgesic

What it's used for: Severe pain from arthritis, surgery or fractures

Dosage: 10 mg every 12 hours (*OxyContin*); 5 mg every 6 hours as needed (*Roxicodone, OxyFAST, OxyIR* [liquid])

Special instructions: Never chew or cut tablets; a potentially fatal dose can occur if the medication is released rapidly. Must be taken whole. Liquid may be mixed with juice, applesauce or pudding.

Possible side effects: Constipation, dizziness, drowsiness, dry mouth, headache, increased sweating, itching of skin, nausea, shortness of breath, vomiting, weakness

Be aware: Over time, this drug may cause psychological and physical dependence. Before taking this drug, let your doctor know if you use a central nervous system depressant, such antihistamines (allergy medications), tranquilizers, sleeping medications, muscle relaxants or narcotic pain medication, or if you have one of the following: liver disease, or history of alcohol or drug abuse.

Oxycodone with acetaminophen

Brand name(s):
Percocet, Endocet

Type of medication: Analgesic

What it's used for: Severe pain from arthritis, surgery or fractures

Dosage: 5 mg oxycodone every 6 hours as needed. (Acetaminophen portion of medication varies, depending on whether you are taking pills or capsules.)

Special instructions: Never chew or cut tablets; a potentially fatal dose can occur if the medication is released rapidly. Must be taken whole.

Possible side effects: Constipation, dizziness, drowsiness, dry mouth, headache, increased sweating, itching of skin, nausea, shortness of breath, vomiting, weakness

Be aware: If you consume 3 or more alcoholic drinks per day, consult your doctor before taking this medication.

Mixing acetaminophen with alcohol can cause liver damage.

Over time, this drug may cause psychological and physical dependence. Before taking this drug, let your doctor know if you use a central nervous system depressant, such as antihistamines (allergy medications), tranquilizers, sleeping medications, muscle relaxants or narcotic pain medications, or if you have one of the following: liver disease, or history of alcohol or drug abuse. Avoid taking more than one product with acetaminophen.

OxyContin

Generic name:
Oxycodone

Other brand name(s):
Roxicodone, OxyFAST, OxyIR (liquid)

Type of medication: Analgesic

What it's used for: Severe pain from arthritis, surgery or fractures

Dosage: 10 mg every 12 hours

Special instructions: Never chew or cut tablets; a potentially fatal dose can occur if the medication is released rapidly. Must be taken whole.

Possible side effects: Constipation, dizziness, drowsiness, dry mouth, headache, increased sweating, itching of skin, nausea, shortness of breath, vomiting, weakness

Be aware: Over time, this drug may cause psychological and physical dependence. Before taking this drug, let your doctor know if you use a central nervous system depressant, such antihistamines (allergy medications), tranquilizers, sleeping medications, muscle relaxants or narcotic pain medication, or if you have one of the following: liver disease, or history of alcohol or drug abuse.

OxyFAST

Generic name:
Oxycodone

Other brand name(s):
OxyContin, Roxicodone, OxyIR (liquid)

Type of medication: Analgesic

What it's used for: Severe pain from arthritis, surgery or fractures

Dosage: 5 mg every 6 hours as needed

Special instructions: Never chew or cut tablets; a potentially fatal dose can occur if the medication is released rapidly. Must be taken whole.

Possible side effects: Constipation, dizziness, drowsiness, dry mouth, headache, increased sweating, itching of skin, nausea, shortness of breath, vomiting, weakness

Be aware: Over time, this drug may cause psychological and physical dependence. Before taking this drug, let your doctor know if you use a central nervous system depressant, such antihistamines (allergy medications), tranquilizers, sleeping medications, muscle relaxants or narcotic pain medication, or if you have one of the following: liver disease, or history of alcohol or drug abuse.

OxyIR (liquid)

Generic name:
Oxycodone

Other brand name(s):
OxyContin, Roxicodone, OxyFAST

Type of medication: Analgesic

What it's used for: Severe pain from arthritis, surgery or fractures

Dosage: 5 mg every 6 hours as needed

Special instructions: Liquid may be mixed with juice, applesauce or pudding.

Possible side effects: Constipation, dizziness, drowsiness, dry mouth, headache, increased sweating, itching of skin, nausea, shortness of breath, vomiting, weakness

Be aware: Over time, this drug may cause psychological and physical dependence. Before taking this drug, let your doctor know if you use a central nervous system depressant, such antihistamines (allergy medications), tranquilizers, sleeping medications, muscle relaxants or narcotic pain medication, or if you have one of the following: liver disease, or history of alcohol or drug abuse.

Panadol

Generic name:
Acetaminophen

Other brand name(s):
Anacin (aspirin-free), Excedrin caplets, Tylenol, Tylenol Arthritis Pain

Type of Medication: Analgesic (OTC)

What it's used for: To relieve pain in any form of arthritis

Dosage: 325 to 1,000 mg every 4 to 6 hours as needed, no more than 4,000 mg per day

Special instructions: Do not use with any other product containing acetaminophen; do not use for more than 10 days for pain – unless directed by a doctor.

Possible side effects: When taken as directed, acetaminophen is usually not associated with side effects.

Be aware: If you consume 3 or more alcoholic drinks per day, consult your doctor before taking acetaminophen. Mixing with alcohol can cause liver damage.

Pediapred

Generic name:

Prednisolone sodium phosphate (liquid only)

Type of medication: Corticosteroid

What it's used for: To control inflammation of joints and organs in many forms of arthritis and related conditions

Dosage: Dosage varies widely according to the disease being treated. Taking either too much or too little can be dangerous. Take exactly the amount prescribed by your doctor.

Special instructions: Take with food. A single daily dose should be taken with breakfast. Sometimes the dose is split, taken 2 to 4 times per day. Don't stop medication abruptly; dosage must be tapered or reduced gradually.

Possible side effects: Bruising, cataracts, elevated blood fats (cholesterol, triglycerides), elevated blood sugar, hardening of the arteries (atherosclerosis), hypertension, increased appetite, indigestion, insomnia, mood swings, muscle weakness, nervousness or restlessness, osteoporosis, susceptibility to infection, thin skin

Be aware: Before taking this medication, let your doctor know if you have one of the following: fungal infection, history of tuberculosis, underactive thyroid, diabetes, stomach ulcer, high blood pressure or osteoporosis.

Penicillamine

Brand name(s):
Cuprimine, Depen

Type of medication: DMARD

What it's used for: Rheumatoid arthritis

Dosage: 125 to 250 mg per day in a single dose to start, increased to not more than 1,500 mg per day in 3 doses

Special instructions: Take on an empty stomach at least 1 hour before or 2 hours after any food, milk or medicine.

Possible side effects: Abdominal pain or upset; diarrhea; flushing; headache; increased sensitivity of the skin to sunlight; itching; joint pain; loss of appetite; nausea or vomiting; skin rash

Be aware: Before taking this medication, let your doctor know if you have any of the following: penicillin allergy, blood disease, kidney disease or lupus. Because this drug can cause blood abnormalities and kidney damage, your doctor should order periodic blood and urine tests to check for unwanted effects. Take consistently; stopping and starting can worsen side effects.

Percocet

Generic name:
Oxycodone with acetaminophen

Type of medication: Analgesic

What it's used for: Severe pain from arthritis, surgery or fractures

Dosage: 5 mg oxycodone every 6 hours as needed. (Acetaminophen portion of medication varies, depending on whether you are taking pills or capsules.)

Special instructions: Never chew or cut tablets; a potentially fatal dose can occur if the medication is released rapidly. Must be taken whole.

Possible side effects: Constipation, dizziness, drowsiness, dry mouth, headache, increased sweating, itching of skin, nausea, shortness of breath, vomiting, weakness

Be aware: If you consume 3 or more alcoholic drinks per day, consult your doctor before taking this medication. Mixing acetaminophen with alcohol can cause liver damage.

Over time, this drug may cause psychological and physical dependence. Before taking this drug, let your doctor know if you use a central nervous system depressant, such as antihistamines (allergy medications), tranquilizers, sleeping medications, muscle relaxants or narcotic pain medications, or if you have one of the following: liver disease, or history of alcohol or drug abuse. Avoid taking more than one product with acetaminophen.

Phenaphen with Codeine

Generic name:
Acetaminophen with Codeine

Other brand name(s):
Tylenol with Codeine #3

Type of medication: Analgesic

What it's used for: Pain not relieved by plain acetaminophen

Dosage: 15 to 60 mg codeine every 4 hours as needed (150 to 600 mg acetaminophen)

Special instructions: Never take more of this drug than your doctor prescribes because high doses of this drug can slow down breathing.

Possible side effects: Constipation, dizziness, lightheadedness, nausea, sedation, shortness of breath, vomiting

Be aware: If you consume 3 or more alcoholic drinks per day, consult your doctor before taking acetaminophen. Mixing this medication with alcohol can cause liver damage. In case of an accidental overdose, contact a physician or poison control center immediately. Over time, this drug may cause psychological and physical dependence. Before taking this drug, let your doctor know if you use central nervous system depressants, such as antihistamines (allergy medications), tranquilizers, sleeping medications, muscle relaxants or narcotic pain medication, or if you have one of the following: liver disease, or history or alcohol or drug abuse. Avoid taking more than one product containing acetaminophen.

Pilocarpine

Brand name(s):
Salagen

Type of medication: Cholinergic agonist

What it's used for: To increase saliva production, relieve dry mouth associated with Sjögren's syndrome

Dosage: 5 to 7.5 mg three to four times per day, not exceeding 30 mg per day

Special instructions: Start with a low dose and take after meals to minimize side effects. Allow 6 to 12 weeks of uninterrupted treatment before improvement is noticed.

Possible side effects: Changes in blood pressure or heart rate; flushing; headache; sweating; urinary frequency

Be aware: Do not take if you have uncontrolled asthma, chronic bronchitis, chronic obstructive pulmonary disease, significant cardiovascular disease, acute iritis or narrow-angle glaucoma. Let your doctor know if you take beta-andrenergic antagonists (beta blockers).

Piroxicam

Brand name(s):
Feldene

Type of medication: NSAID

What it's used for: To ease arthritis pain and inflammation

Dosage: 20 mg per day in 1 or 2 doses

Special instructions: Do not take with other prescription or OTC NSAIDs. Take as directed at the same time(s) every day. If you experience stomach upset, take with food, a glass of milk or an antacid.

Possible side effects: Abdominal or stomach cramps, pain or discomfort; diarrhea; dizziness; edema (swelling of the feet); headache; gastrointestinal bleeding; heartburn or indigestion; nausea or vomiting; peptic ulcer

Be aware: Before taking this medication, let your doctor know if you drink alcohol or use blood thinners, or if you have or have had any of the following: sensitivity or allergy to aspirin or similar drugs, kidney or liver disease, heart disease, high blood pressure, asthma or stomach ulcers. Because stomach ulcers or internal bleeding can occur without warning, regular checkups are important. Patients on long-term NSAIDs should have blood counts and liver enzymes checked periodically.

Unlike low-dose aspirin, there is little evidence that this or other NSAIDs will protect against heart attack or stroke. NSAIDs may be used with low-dose aspirin, but doing so may slightly increase your risk of gastric bleeding. Before taking this or any NSAID, tell your doctor if you take ACE inhibitors, lithium, warfarin or furosemide.

All NSAIDs may cause an increased risk of serious blood clots, heart attacks and stroke, which can be fatal. This risk may increase with dose and duration of use. Patients with cardiovascular disease or risk factors for cardiovascular disease may be at higher risk. These drugs should not be used for pain in people having coronary bypass surgery.

Plaquenil

Generic name:
Hydroxychloroquine sulfate

Type of medication: DMARD

What it's used for: Rheumatoid arthritis, lupus

Dosage: 200 to 600 mg per day in 1 or 2 doses

Possible side effects: Blurred vision; diarrhea; headache; increased sensitivity to sunlight; itching; loss of appetite; nausea or vomiting; rashes; stomach cramps or pain

Be aware: Let your doctor know if you have any eye problems, including a retinal abnormality. Because vision may be damaged with long-term therapy (given over several years), you may need to have an eye exam when you start taking the drug and every 6 to 12 months thereafter to detect retinal changes.

Ponstel

Generic name:
Mefenamic acid

Type of medication: NSAID

What it's used for: To ease arthritis pain and inflammation

Dosage: 500 mg initial dose, then 250 mg every 6 hours as needed, for up to 7 days

Special instructions: Do not take with other prescription or OTC NSAIDs. Take as directed at the same time(s) every day. If you experience stomach upset, take with food or a glass of milk.

Possible side effects: Abdominal or stomach cramps, pain or discomfort; diarrhea; dizziness; edema (swelling of the feet); headache; gastrointestinal bleeding; heartburn or indigestion; nausea or vomiting; peptic ulcer

Be aware: Before taking this medication, let your doctor know if you drink alcohol or use blood thinners or if you have or have had any of the following: sensitivity or allergy to aspirin or similar drugs, kidney or liver disease, heart disease, high blood pressure, asthma or stomach ulcers. Because stomach ulcers or internal bleeding can occur without warning, regular checkups are important.

Unlike low-dose aspirin, there is little evidence that this or other NSAIDs will protect against heart attack or stroke. NSAIDs may be used with low-dose aspirin, but doing so may slightly increase your risk of gastric bleeding. Before taking this or any NSAID, tell your doctor if you take ACE inhibitors, lithium, warfarin or furosemide.

This medication is for short-term relief of pain and should not be used for more than 7 days.

All NSAIDs may cause an increased risk of serious blood clots, heart attacks and stroke, which can be fatal. This risk may increase with dose and duration of use. Patients with cardiovascular disease or risk factors for cardiovascular disease may be at higher risk. These drugs should not be used for pain in people having coronary bypass surgery.

PP-Cap

Generic name:
Propoxyphene hydrochloride

Other brand name(s):
Darvon

Type of medication: Analgesic

What it's used for: Severe pain from arthritis, surgery or fractures

Dosage: 65 mg every 4 hours as needed, no more than 390 mg per day

Special instructions: Never take more of this drug than your doctor prescribes. Do not increase dose on your own because side effects increase and tolerance develops as dosage increases. Do not drive or operate heavy machinery until you know how your body reacts to this drug.

Possible side effects: Dizziness, nausea, sedation, vomiting

Be aware: Over time, this drug may cause psychological and physical dependence. Before taking this drug, let your doctor know if you use a central nervous system depressant, such as antihistamines (allergy medications), tranquilizers, sleeping medications, muscle relaxants or narcotic pain medications, or if you have one of the following: liver disease, or history of alcohol or drug abuse.

Prednicen-M

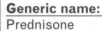

Generic name:
Prednisone

Other brand name(s):
Deltasone, Orasone, Sterapred

Type of medication: Corticosteroid

What it's used for: To control inflammation of joints and organs in many forms of arthritis and related conditions

Dosage: Dosage varies widely according to the disease being treated. Taking either too much or too little can be dangerous. Take exactly the amount prescribed by your doctor.

Special instructions: Take with food. A single daily dose should be taken with breakfast. Sometimes the dose is split, taken 2 to 4 times per day. Don't stop medication abruptly; dosage must be tapered or reduced gradually.

Possible side effects: Bruising, cataracts, elevated blood fats (cholesterol, triglycerides), elevated blood sugar, hard-

ening of the arteries (atherosclerosis), hypertension, increased appetite, indigestion, insomnia, mood swings, muscle weakness, nervousness or restlessness, osteoporosis, susceptibility to infection, thin skin

Be aware: Before taking this medication, let your doctor know if you have one of the following: fungal infection, history of tuberculosis, underactive thyroid, diabetes, stomach ulcer, high blood pressure or osteoporosis.

Prednisolone

Brand name(s):
Prelone

Type of medication: Corticosteroid

What it's used for: To control inflammation of joints and organs in many forms of arthritis and related conditions

Dosage: Dosage varies widely according to the disease being treated. Taking either too much or too little can be dangerous. Take exactly the amount prescribed by your doctor.

Special instructions: Take with food. A single daily dose should be taken with breakfast. Sometimes the dose is split, taken 2 to 4 times per day. Don't stop medication abruptly; dosage must be tapered or reduced gradually.

Possible side effects: Bruising, cataracts, elevated blood fats (cholesterol, triglycerides), elevated blood sugar, hard-

ening of the arteries (atherosclerosis), hypertension, increased appetite, indigestion, insomnia, mood swings, muscle weakness, nervousness or restlessness, osteoporosis, susceptibility to infection, thin skin

Be aware: Before taking this medication, let your doctor know if you have one of the following: fungal infection, history of tuberculosis, underactive thyroid, diabetes, stomach ulcer, high blood pressure or osteoporosis.

Prednisolone sodium phosphate

(liquid only)

Brand name(s):
Pediapred

Type of medication: Corticosteroid

What it's used for: To control inflammation of joints and organs in many forms of arthritis and related conditions

Dosage: Dosage varies widely according to the disease being treated. Taking either too much or too little can be dangerous. Take exactly the amount prescribed by your doctor.

Special instructions: Take with food. A single daily dose should be taken with breakfast. Sometimes the dose is split, taken 2 to 4 times per day. Don't stop medication abruptly; dosage must be tapered or reduced gradually.

Possible side effects: Bruising, cataracts, elevated blood fats (cholesterol, triglycerides), elevated blood sugar, hard-

ening of the arteries (atherosclerosis), hypertension, increased appetite, indigestion, insomnia, mood swings, muscle weakness, nervousness or restlessness, osteoporosis, susceptibility to infection, thin skin

Be aware: Before taking this medication, let your doctor know if you have one of the following: fungal infection, history of tuberculosis, underactive thyroid, diabetes, stomach ulcer, high blood pressure or osteoporosis.

Prednisone

Brand name(s):
Deltasone, Orasone, Prednicen-M, Sterapred

Type of medication: Corticosteroid

What it's used for: To control inflammation of joints and organs in many forms of arthritis and related conditions

Dosage: Dosage varies widely according to the disease being treated. Taking either too much or too little can be dangerous. Take exactly the amount prescribed by your doctor.

Special instructions: Take with food. A single daily dose should be taken with breakfast. Sometimes the dose is split, taken 2 to 4 times per day. Don't stop medication abruptly; dosage must be tapered or reduced gradually.

Possible side effects: Bruising, cataracts, elevated blood fats (cholesterol, triglycerides), elevated blood sugar, hardening of the arteries (atherosclerosis), hypertension, increased appetite, indigestion, insomnia, mood swings, muscle weakness, nervousness or restlessness, osteoporosis, susceptibility to infection, thin skin

Be aware: Before taking this medication, let your doctor know if you have one of the following: fungal infection, history of tuberculosis, underactive thyroid, diabetes, stomach ulcer, high blood pressure or osteoporosis.

Prelone

Generic name:
Prednisolone

Type of medication: Corticosteroid

What it's used for: To control inflammation of joints and organs in many forms of arthritis and related conditions

Dosage: Dosage varies widely according to the disease being treated. Taking either too much or too little can be dangerous. Take exactly the amount prescribed by your doctor.

Special instructions: Take with food. A single daily dose should be taken with breakfast. Sometimes the dose is split, taken 2 to 4 times per day. Don't stop medication abruptly; dosage must be tapered or reduced gradually.

Possible side effects: Bruising, cataracts, elevated blood fats (cholesterol, triglycerides), elevated blood sugar, hardening of the arteries (atherosclerosis), hypertension, increased appetite, indigestion, insomnia, mood swings, muscle weakness, nervousness or restlessness, osteoporosis, susceptibility to infection, thin skin

Be aware: Before taking this medication, let your doctor know if you have one of the following: fungal infection, history of tuberculosis, underactive thyroid, diabetes, stomach ulcer, high blood pressure or osteoporosis.

Premarin, see Estrogens
(without progesterone)

Premphase, see Estrogens
(with progesterone)

Prempro, see Estrogens
(with progesterone)

Probalan

Generic name:
Probenecid

Other brand name(s):
Benemid

Type of medication: Uric-acid-lowering medication

What it's used for: To reduce uric acid and decrease the frequency and severity of gout attacks

Dosage: 500 to 3,000 mg per day in 2 or 3 divided doses

Special instructions: Take with food or an antacid. Do not take with aspirin or other NSAIDs. Avoid alcohol.

Possible side effects: Headache, loss of appetite, nausea or vomiting

Be aware: This drug may interfere with the copper sulfate urine sugar tests taken by people with diabetes and lead to false positive readings.

Proben-C, see Probenecid and colchicine

Probenecid

Brand name(s):
Benemid, Probalan

Type of medication: Uric-acid-lowering medication

What it's used for: To reduce uric acid and decrease the frequency and severity of gout attacks

Dosage: 500 to 3,000 mg per day in 2 or 3 divided doses

Special instructions: Take with food or an antacid. Do not take with aspirin or other NSAIDs. Avoid alcohol.

Possible side effects: Headache, worsening of gout, loss of appetite, nausea or vomiting

Be aware: This drug may interfere with the copper sulfate urine sugar tests taken by people with diabetes and lead to false-positive readings.

Probenecid and colchicine

Brand name(s):
ColBenemid, Col-Probenecid, Proben-C

Type of medication: Gout medication

What it's used for: To increase excretion of uric acid and control inflammation of gout attacks

Dosage: 1 tablet (500 mg probenecid and 0.5 mg colchicine) 2 times per day

Special instructions: Take with food or an antacid. Drink plenty of fluids. Do not take with aspirin or other NSAIDs. Avoid alcohol.

Possible side effects: Diarrhea, headache, loss of appetite, nausea or vomiting, stomach pain

Be aware: Before taking this drug, tell your doctor if you use cancer medications, heparin (*Calciparine, Liquaemin*), nitrofuratoin (*Furadantin, Macrobid, Macrodantin*), NSAIDs or zidovudine (*Retrovir*), or if you have any of the following: blood disease, intestinal disease, kidney disease or kidney stones.

Propoxyphene hydrochloride

Brand name(s):
Darvon, PP-Cap

Type of medication: Analgesic

What it's used for: Severe pain from arthritis, surgery or fractures

Dosage: 65 mg every 4 hours as needed, no more than 390 mg per day

Special instructions: Never take more of this drug than your doctor prescribes. Do not increase dose on your own because side effects increase and tolerance develops as dosage increases; do not drive or operate heavy machinery until you know how your body reacts to this drug.

Possible side effects: Dizziness, nausea, sedation, vomiting

Be aware: Over time, this drug may cause psychological and physical dependence. Before taking this drug, let your doctor know if you use a central nervous system depressant, such as antihistamines (allergy medications), tranquilizers, sleeping medications, muscle relaxants or narcotic pain medications, or if you have one of the following: liver disease, or history of alcohol or drug abuse.

Propoxyphene with acetaminophen

Brand name(s):
Darvocet

Type of medication: Analgesic

What it's used for: Severe pain from arthritis, surgery or fractures

Dosage: 50 to 100 mg propoxyphene (325 to 650 mg acetaminophen) every 4 hours as needed, not to exceed 600 mg propoxyphene per day

Special instructions: Never take more of this drug than your doctor prescribes. Do not increase dose on your own because side effects increase and tolerance develops as dosage increases; do not drive or operate heavy machinery until you know how your body reacts to this drug.

Possible side effects: Dizziness, nausea, sedation, vomiting

Be aware: If you consume 3 or more alcoholic drinks per day, consult your doctor before taking this medication. Mixing acetaminophen with alcohol can cause liver damage.

Over time, this drug may cause psychological and physical dependence. Before taking this drug, let your doctor know if you use a central nervous system depressant, such as antihistamines (allergy medications), tranquilizers, sleeping medications, muscle relaxants or narcotic pain medications, or if you have one of the following: liver disease, or history of alcohol or drug abuse.

Prozac

Generic name:

Fluoxetine

Type of medication: Antidepressant (SSRI)

What it's used for: To improve depression, relieve fatigue and improve energy in people with fibromyalgia

Dosage: 20 to 80 mg per day in a single dose

Special instructions: Build dose gradually; taper dose slowly.

Possible side effects: Anxiety or nervousness; constipation; decrease in sexual desire or ability; decreased appetite; diarrhea; drowsiness; dry mouth; headache; hives or itching; increased sweating; nausea; restlessness; skin rash; tiredness or weakness; trembling or shaking; trouble sleeping. Side effects may continue after treatment is stopped.

Be aware: Combining this drug with alcohol or other central nervous system depressants (including antihistamines, narcotic medications and some dental anesthetics) can increase their effects and side effects. Taking with aspirin or other NSAIDs may increase risk of bleeding. Never stop taking this medication abruptly. Your doctor will taper your dosage gradually. Do not take within 14 days of taking a monoamine oxidase (MAO) inhibitor. Patients and their family members should be aware of agitation and suicidal tendencies.

R-u

Raloxifene hydrochloride

Brand name(s):
Evista

Type of medication: Selective estrogen receptor molecule (SERM)

What it's used for: Osteoporosis

Dosage: 60 mg per day in a single dose

Special instructions: Take any time of day with or without food.

Possible side effects: Blood clots in veins; hot flashes, leg cramps

Be aware: This drug should not be used prior to menopause. Let your doctor know if there is a chance you could be pregnant or if you have a history of blood clots or if you use cholestyramine or warfarin (*Coumadin*).

Relafen

Generic name:
Nabumetone

Type of medication: NSAID

What it's used for: To ease arthritis pain and inflammation

Dosage: 1,000 mg per day in 1 or 2 doses; 2,000 mg per day in 2 doses

Special instructions: Do not take with other prescription or OTC NSAIDs. Take as directed at the same time(s) every day. If you experience stomach upset, take with food, a glass of milk or an antacid.

Possible side effects: Abdominal or stomach cramps, pain or discomfort; diarrhea; dizziness; edema (swelling of the feet); gastrointestinal bleeding; headache; heartburn or indigestion; nausea or vomiting; peptic ulcer

Be aware: Before taking this medication, let your doctor know if you drink alcohol or use blood thinners, or if you have or have had any of the following: sensitivity or allergy to aspirin or similar drugs, kidney or liver disease, heart disease, high blood pressure, asthma or stomach ulcers. Because stomach ulcers or internal bleeding can occur without warning, regular checkups are important. Patients on long term NSAIDs should have blood counts and liver enzymes checked periodically.

Unlike low-dose aspirin, there is little evidence that this or other NSAIDs will protect against heart attack or stroke. NSAIDs may be used with low-dose aspirin, but doing so may slightly increase your risk of gastric bleeding. Before taking this or any NSAID, tell your doctor if you take ACE inhibitors, lithium, warfarin or furosemide.

All NSAIDs may cause an increased risk of serious blood clots, heart attacks and stroke, which can be fatal. This risk may increase with dose and duration of use. Patients with cardiovascular disease or risk factors for cardiovascular disease may be at higher risk. These drugs should not be used for pain in people having coronary bypass surgery.

Remicade

Generic name:
Infliximab

Type of medication: Biologic response modifier

What it's used for: To control symptoms, prevent joint damage and improve physical function in rheumatoid arthritis, psoriatic arthritis and ankylosing spondylitis

Dosage: Dose is based on body weight and ranges from 200 mg to 400 mg per treatment for most patients. After three initial infusions at 0, 2 and 6 weeks, infusions are repeated every 8 weeks.

Special instructions: Drug is infused intravenously (IV) during a 2-hour infusion done in a doctor's office, clinic or hospital. Patients taking infliximab should also be taking methotrexate once a week by mouth or injection.

Possible side effects: Infusion reactions (occurring during or shortly after the infusion) including chest pain, change in blood pressure, difficulty breathing and hives; redness and pain; itching, swelling and/or bruising at the injection site; upper respiratory infection

Be aware: Rheumatoid arthritis carries a higher risk of infection and lymphoma. It is uncertain whether this and other biologic response modifiers increase lymphoma risk. Discontinue if you have a serious infection (such as pneumonia) or recurrent infections. Live vaccines should not be given along with this drug, but the flu vaccine or the vaccine for pneumonia (*Pneumovax*) can be safely given.

Let your doctor know if you have a history of (or currently have) one of the following: active infection, recurrent infection, exposure to tuberculosis or positive skin test for tuberculosis; or if you have a nervous system disorder, including neurological disorders such as multiple sclerosis, seizure disorders, myelitis or optic neuritis.

Patients with congestive heart failure (CHF) should not be given this drug.

Rarely, a lupus-like syndrome may develop, with symptoms such as rash, fever and pleurisy, which may resolve when medication is stopped. Multiple sclerosis, has rarely developed in patients receiving this drug or etanercept.

Infusion reaction may be treated by slowing the speed of infusion as well as by pre-treatment with acetaminophen, antihistamine (*Benadryl, Claritin*) or steroid medication (hydrocortisone, prednisone).

Restasis

Generic name:
Cyclosporine ophthalmic emulsion

Type of medication: Immunosuppressive/eye drop

What it's used for: To relieve dry eyes associated with Sjögren's syndrome

Dosage: One drop in each eye twice per day, approximately 12 hours apart

Special instructions: Single-use vials must be used immediately upon opening and then discarded.

Possible side effects: Blurred vision; burning, pain, itching or stinging feelings in eye; discharge; foreign body sensation

Be aware: Cyclosporine is an immunosuppressant. Do not use if you have an eye infection. Do not wear contact lenses while using this medication.

Rheumatrex

Generic name:
Methotrexate

Other brand name(s):
Trexall

Type of medication: DMARD

What it's used for: Rheumatoid arthritis, lupus, and other forms of arthritis

Dosage: 7.5 to 20 mg per week in a single dose orally (This drug may also be given by injection.)

Possible side effects: Abdominal discomfort, chills, dizziness, fever, general feeling of illness, hair loss, headache, increased sun sensitivity, itching, liver problems, low blood counts, mouth sores, nausea and stomach upset, rashes, shortness of breath, yeast infection

Be aware: Let your doctor know if you have one of the following: abnormal blood count, liver or lung disease, alcoholism, active infection or hepatitis. Your doctor should order chest X-rays, liver tests and blood counts before you start this drug and throughout treatment to monitor for side effects. Alert your doctor immediately if you have a dry cough, fever or difficulty breathing. This drug can rarely be associated with increased risk of blood diseases such as lymphoma.

Ridaura

Generic name:
Auranofin (oral gold)

Type of medication: DMARD

What it's used for: Rheumatoid arthritis

Dosage: 6 to 9 mg per day in 1 or 2 doses

Special instructions: Take with a glass of milk or water. If stomach upset occurs, take with food.

Possible side effects: Diarrhea, low blood counts, metallic taste in mouth, mouth ulcers, protein in urine, skin rash or itching

Be aware: Before taking this drug, let your doctor know if you have or have had one of the following: adverse reaction to a gold-containing medication, a history of blood-cell abnormality, inflammatory bowel disease, or kidney or liver disease. This drug can cause sun sensitivity, so minimize exposure to sunlight and sunlamps and wear sunscreen when outdoors. Your doctor should order periodic blood and urine tests to check for effects on the blood and kidneys.

Risedronate sodium

Brand name(s):
Actonel

Type of medication: Bisphosphonate

What it's used for: Treatment or prevention of osteoporosis

Dosage: 5 mg per day in a single dose or 35 mg per week in a single dose

Special instructions: Take only with 1 cup of water first thing in the morning. Swallow pill whole while sitting or standing and stay upright for 30 minutes.

Possible side effects: Abdominal or stomach pain, heartburn

Be aware: Before taking this medication, let your doctor know if you are taking aspirin or aspirin-containing products or if you have problems with the esophagus, stomach or kidneys. Blood levels of calcium and vitamin D must be normal before starting therapy.

Risedronate with calcium

Brand name:
Actonel with calcium

Type of medication: Bisphosphonate with calcium supplement

What it's used for: osteoporosis treatment and prevention

Dosage: Risedronate is taken in a single weekly dose of 35 mg; calcium tables taken other six days

Special instructions: Risedronate sodium: Take only with water in the morning. Swallow pill whole while sitting or standing; stay upright; avoid food for 30 minutes. Calcium tablets: Take with food.

Possible side effects: Abdominal or stomach pain; heartburn

Be aware: Before taking this medication, let your doctor know if you are taking aspirin or aspirin-containing products, or if you have problems with the esophagus, stomach or kidneys. Blood levels of calcium and vitamin D must be normal before starting therapy.

Rituxan

Generic name:
Rituximab

Type of medication: Biologic response modifier

What it's used for: Moderately to severely active rheumatoid arthritis that hasn't responded to other biologic response modifiers

Dosage: Two 1000-mg doses given two weeks apart

Special instructions: Drug is infused intravenously (IV) in doctor's office, clinic or hospital. Intravenous corticosteroids should be administered 30 minutes prior to the infusion to reduce the incidence and severity of infusion reactions.

Possible side effects: Abdominal pain, anxiety, chills, fever, headache, high cholesterol, hives, hypertension, itching, joint pain, nausea, sore throat, stomach upset, upper respiratory infection, weakness

Be aware: Discontinue if you have a serious or recurrent infection. Do not take live vaccines; the pneumonia vaccine (*Pneumovax*) or flu vaccine can be safely given. Let your doctor know if you have or are a carrier for hepatitis b or if you have heart or lung disease.

Rituximab

Brand name:
Rituxan

Type of medication: Biologic response modifier

What it's used for: Moderately to severely active rheumatoid arthritis that hasn't responded to other biologic response modifiers

Dosage: Two 1000-mg doses given two weeks apart

Special instructions: Drug is infused intravenously (IV) in doctor's office, clinic or hospital. Intravenous corticosteroids should be administered 30 minutes prior to the infusion to reduce the incidence and severity of infusion reactions.

Possible side effects: Abdominal pain, anxiety, chills, fever, headache, high cholesterol, hives, hypertension, itching, joint pain, nausea, sore throat, stomach upset, upper respiratory infection, weakness

Be aware: Discontinue if you have a serious or recurrent infection. Do not take live vaccines; the pneumonia vaccine (*Pneumovax*) or flu vaccine can be safely given. Let your doctor know if you have or are a carrier for hepatitis B or if you have heart or lung disease.

Roxicodone

Generic name:
Oxycodone

Other brand name(s):
OxyContin, OxyFAST, OxyIR (liquid)

Type of medication: Analgesic

What it's used for: Severe pain from arthritis, surgery or fractures

Dosage: 5 mg every 6 hours as needed

Special instructions: Never chew or cut tablets; a potentially fatal dose can be administered if medication is released rapidly. Must be taken whole.

Possible side effects: Constipation, dizziness, drowsiness, dry mouth, headache, increased sweating, itching of skin, nausea, shortness of breath, vomiting, weakness

Be aware: Over time, this drug may cause psychological and physical dependence. Before taking this drug, let your doctor know if you use a central nervous system depressant, such antihistamines (allergy medications), tranquilizers, sleeping medications, muscle relaxants or narcotic pain medication, or if you have one of the following: liver disease, or history of alcohol or drug abuse.

Salagen

Generic name:
Pilocarpine

Type of medication: Cholinergic agonist

What it's used for: To increase saliva production, relieve dry mouth associated with Sjögren's syndrome

Dosage: 5 to 7.5 mg three to four times per day, not exceeding 30 mg per day

Special instructions: Start with a low dose and take after meals to minimize side effects. Allow 6 to 12 weeks of uninterrupted treatment before improvement is noticed.

Possible side effects: Changes in blood pressure or heart rate; flushing; headache; sweating; urinary frequency

Be aware: Do not take if you have uncontrolled asthma, chronic bronchitis, chronic obstructive pulmonary disease, significant cardiovascular disease, acute iritis or narrow-angle glaucoma. Let your doctor know if ou take beta-andrenergic antagonists (beta blockers).

Salflex, see Salsalate

Salsalate

Brand name(s):

Amigesic, Anaflex 750, Disalcid, Marthritic, Mono-Gesic, Salflex, Salsitab

Type of medication: NSAID (nonacetylated salicylate)

What it's used for: To ease arthritis pain and inflammation

Dosage: 1,000 to 3,000 mg per day in 2 or 3 doses

Special instructions: Take with food. Do not chew tablets. Do not crush enteric-coated or time-release forms and mix with water. Do not combine with other NSAIDs.

Possible side effects: Abdominal or stomach cramps, pain or discomfort; diarrhea; dizziness; edema (swelling of the feet); gastrointestinal bleeding; headache; heartburn or indigestion; nausea or vomiting; peptic ulcer

Be aware: Dizziness, deafness or ringing in the ears indicates that you are taking too much. Before taking these medications, let your doctor know if you drink alcohol or use other NSAIDs. If you are taking doses of more than 3,600 mg per day, your doctor should monitor salicylate levels in your blood.

Salsitab, see Salsalate

Sodium salicylate

Brand name(s):
Available as generic only

Type of medication: NSAID (nonacetylated salicylate)

What it's used for: To ease arthritis pain and inflammation

Dosage: 3,600 to 5,400 mg per day in several doses

Special instructions: Take with food. Do not chew tablets. Do not crush enteric-coated or time-release forms and mix with water. Do not combine with other NSAIDs.

Possible side effects: Abdominal or stomach cramps, pain or discomfort; diarrhea; dizziness or lightheadedness; edema (swelling of the feet); headache; heartburn or indigestion; nausea or vomiting

Be aware: Dizziness, deafness or ringing in the ears indicates that you are taking too much. Before taking this medication, let your doctor know if you drink alcohol or use other NSAIDs. If you are taking doses of more than 3,600 mg per day, your doctor should monitor salicylate levels in your blood.

Sterapred

Generic name:
Prednisone

Other brand name(s):
Deltasone, Orasone, Prednicen-M

Type of medication: Corticosteroid

What it's used for: To control inflammation of joints and organs in many forms of arthritis and related conditions

Dosage: Dosage varies widely according to the disease being treated. Taking either too much or too little can be dangerous. Take exactly the amount prescribed by your doctor.

Special instructions: Take with food. A single daily dose should be taken with breakfast. Sometimes the dose is split, taken 2 to 4 times per day. Don't stop medication abruptly; dosage must be tapered or reduced gradually.

Possible side effects: Bruising, cataracts, elevated blood fats (cholesterol, triglycerides), elevated blood sugar, hardening of the arteries (atherosclerosis), hypertension, increased appetite, indigestion, insomnia, mood swings, muscle weakness, nervousness or restlessness, osteoporosis, susceptibility to infection, thin skin

Be aware: Before taking this medication, let your doctor know if you have one of the following: fungal infection, history of tuberculosis, underactive thyroid, diabetes, stomach ulcer, high blood pressure or osteoporosis.

Sulfasalazine

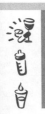

Brand name(s):
Azulfidine, Azulfidine EN-Tabs

Type of medication: DMARD

What it's used for: Rheumatoid arthritis, lupus, ankylosing spondylitis and other forms of arthritis

Dosage: 500 to 3,000 mg per day in 2 to 4 doses

Possible side effects: Abdominal or stomach pain or upset, aching of joints, diarrhea, headache, increased sensitivity of skin to sunlight, itching, loss of appetite, nausea or vomiting, skin rash

Be aware: Before taking this medication, let your doctor know if you have any of the following: allergy to sulfa drugs or aspirin; kidney, liver or blood disease. Failure to drink adequate fluids while on this medication can lead to the formation of urine crystals. This drug can lower sperm counts in men and may interfere with the ability to conceive. Your doctor should order periodic blood tests to check for side effects of this drug.

Sulindac

Brand name(s):
Clinoril

Type of medication: NSAID

What it's used for: To ease arthritis pain and inflammation

Dosage: 300 to 400 mg per day in 2 doses

Special instructions: Do not take with other prescription or OTC NSAIDs. Take as directed at the same time(s) every day. If you experience stomach upset, take with food, a glass of milk or an antacid.

Possible side effects: Abdominal or stomach cramps, pain or discomfort; diarrhea; dizziness; edema (swelling of the feet); headache; gastrointestinal bleeding; heartburn or indigestion; nausea or vomiting; peptic ulcer

Be aware: Before taking this medication, let your doctor know if you drink alcohol or use blood thinners, or if you have or have had any of the following: sensitivity or allergy to aspirin or similar drugs, kidney or liver disease, heart disease, high blood pressure, asthma or stomach ulcers. Because stomach ulcers or internal bleeding can occur without warning, regular checkups are important. Patients on long-term NSAIDs should have blood counts and liver enzymes checked periodically.

Unlike low-dose aspirin, there is little evidence that this or other NSAIDs will protect against heart attack or stroke. NSAIDs may be used with low-dose aspirin, but doing so may slightly increase your risk of gastric bleeding. Before taking this or any NSAID, tell your doctor if you take ACE inhibitors, lithium, warfarin or furosemide.

All NSAIDs may cause an increased risk of serious blood clots, heart attacks and stroke, which can be fatal. This risk may increase with dose and duration of use. Patients with cardiovascular disease or risk factors for cardiovascular disease may be at higher risk. These drugs should not be used for pain in people having coronary bypass surgery.

Teriparatide

Brand name(s):
Forteo

Type of medication: Bone formation agent

What it's used for: Osteoporosis

Dosage: 20 micrograms (mcg) per day in a single dose

Special instructions: Inject into the abdomen or thigh using multidose, prefilled pen delivery device provided by the manufacturer.

Possible side effects: Dizziness, leg cramps

Be aware: Do not take this drug if you have ever had bone cancer or radiation or if you have high levels of calcium in your blood. Urinary excretion of calcium should be monitored if you have urinary tract stones or a high calcium level.

Tolectin, see tolmetin sodium

Tolmetin sodium

Brand name(s):
Tolectin

Type of medication: NSAID

What it's used for: To ease arthritis pain and inflammation

Dosage: 1,200 to 1,800 mg per day in 3 doses

Special instructions: Do not take with other prescription or OTC NSAIDs. Take as directed at the same time(s) every day. If you experience stomach upset, take with food, a glass of milk or an antacid.

Possible side effects: Abdominal or stomach cramps, pain or discomfort; diarrhea; dizziness; edema (swelling of the feet); gastrointestinal bleeding; headache; heartburn or indigestion; nausea or vomiting; peptic ulcer

Be aware: Before taking this medication, let your doctor know if you drink alcohol or use blood thinners, or if you have or have had any of the following: sensitivity or allergy to aspirin or similar drugs, kidney or liver disease, heart disease, high blood pressure, asthma or stomach ulcers. Because stomach ulcers or internal bleeding can occur without warning, regular checkups are important. Patients on long-term NSAIDs should have blood counts and liver enzymes checked periodically.

Unlike low-dose aspirin, there is little evidence that this or other NSAIDs will protect against heart attack or stroke. NSAIDs may be used with low-dose aspirin, but doing so may slightly increase your risk of gastric bleeding. Before taking this or any NSAID, tell your doctor if you take ACE inhibitors, lithium, warfarin or furosemide.

All NSAIDs may cause an increased risk of serious blood clots, heart attacks and stroke, which can be fatal. This risk may increase with dose and duration of use. Patients with cardiovascular disease or risk factors for cardiovascular disease may be at higher risk. These drugs should not be used for pain in people having coronary bypass surgery.

Tramadol

Brand name(s):
Ultram

Type of medication: Analgesic

What it's used for: Severe pain from arthritis, fibromyalgia, surgery or fractures

Dosage: 50 to 100 mg every 4 to 6 hours as needed

Special instructions: Do not increase your dose on your own; do not stop abruptly unless advised to do so by your doctor; do not drive or operate heavy machinery until you know how your body reacts to this drug.

Possible side effects: Constipation, diarrhea, dizziness, drowsiness, increased sweating, loss of appetite, nausea

Be aware: Over time, this drug may cause psychological and physical dependence. Before taking this drug, let your doctor know if you use a central nervous system depressant, such as antihistamines (allergy medications), tranquilizers, sleeping medications, muscle relaxants or narcotic pain medications, or if you have one of the following: liver disease, or history of alcohol or drug abuse.

Tramadol with acetaminophen

Brand name(s):
Ultracet

Type of medication: Analgesic

What it's used for: Severe pain from arthritis, fibromyalgia, surgery or fractures

Dosage: 75 mg tramadol every 4 to 6 hours as needed for up to 5 days (no more than 600 mg per day)

Special instructions: Do not increase your dose on your own; do not stop abruptly unless advised to do so by your doctor. Do not take with other medications containing acetaminophen. Do not drive or operate heavy machinery until you know how your body reacts to this drug.

Possible side effects: Constipation, diarrhea, dizziness, drowsiness, increased sweating, loss of appetite, nausea

Be aware: If you consume 3 or more alcoholic drinks per day, consult your doctor before taking this medication. Mixing acetaminophen with alcohol can cause liver damage. In case of accidental overdose, contact a physician or poison control center immediately.

Over time, this drug may cause psychological and physical dependence. Before taking this drug, let your doctor know if you use a central nervous system depressant, such as antihistamines (allergy medications), tranquilizers, sleeping medications, muscle relaxants or narcotic pain medications, or if you have one of the following: liver disease, or history of alcohol or drug abuse. Avoid taking more than one product containing acetaminophen.

Trexall

Generic name:
Methotrexate

Other brand name(s):
Rheumatrex

Type of medication: DMARD

What it's used for: Rheumatoid arthritis, lupus and other forms of arthritis

Dosage: 7.5 to 20 mg per week in a single dose orally (this drug may also be given by injection)

Possible side effects: Abdominal discomfort, chills, dizziness, fever, general feeling of illness, hair loss, headache, increased sun sensitivity, itching, liver problems, low blood counts, mouth sores, nausea and stomach upset, rashes, shortness of breath, sleepiness, weakness

Be aware: Let your doctor know if you have one of the following: abnormal blood count, liver or lung disease, alcoholism, active infection or hepatitis. Your doctor should order chest X-rays, liver tests and blood counts before you start this drug and throughout treatment to monitor for side effects. Alert your doctor immediately if you have a dry cough, fever or difficulty breathing. This drug can rarely be associated with increased risk of blood diseases such as lymphoma.

Tricosal

Generic name:
Choline and magnesium salicylates

Other brand name(s):
CMT, Trilisate

Type of medication: NSAID (nonacetylated salicylate)

What it's used for: To ease arthritis pain and inflammation

Dosage: 2,000 to 3,000 mg per day in 2 or 3 doses

Special instructions: Take with food. Do not chew tablets. Do not crush enteric-coated or time-release forms and mix with water. Do not combine with other NSAIDs.

Possible side effects: Abdominal or stomach cramps, pain or discomfort; diarrhea; dizziness or lightheadedness; edema (swelling of the feet); headache; heartburn or indigestion; nausea or vomiting

Be aware: Dizziness, deafness or ringing in the ears indicates that you are taking too much. Before taking this medication, let your doctor know if you drink alcohol or use other NSAIDs. If you are taking doses of more than 3,600 mg per day, your doctor should monitor salicylate levels in your blood.

Trilisate

Generic name:
Choline and magnesium salicylates

Other brand name(s):
CMT, Tricosal

Type of medication: NSAID (nonacetylated salicylate)

What it's used for: To ease arthritis pain and inflammation

Dosage: 2,000 to 3,000 mg per day in 2 or 3 doses

Special instructions: Take with food. Do not chew tablets. Do not crush enteric-coated or time-release forms and mix with water. Do not combine with other NSAIDs.

Possible side effects: Abdominal or stomach cramps, pain or discomfort; diarrhea; dizziness or lightheadedness; edema (swelling of the feet); headache; heartburn or indigestion; nausea or vomiting

Be aware: Dizziness, deafness or ringing in the ears indicates that you are taking too much. Before taking this medication, let your doctor know if you drink alcohol or use other NSAIDs. If you are taking doses of more than 3,600 mg per day, your doctor should monitor salicylate levels in your blood.

Tylenol

Generic name:
Acetaminophen

Other brand name(s):
Anacin (aspirin-free), Excedrin caplets, Panadol,
Tylenol Arthritis Pain

Type of Medication: Analgesic (OTC)

What it's used for: To relieve pain in any form of arthritis

Dosage: 325 to 1,000 mg every 4 to 6 hours as needed, no more than 4,000 mg per day

Special instructions: Do not use with any other product containing acetaminophen; do not use for more than 10 days for pain – unless directed by a doctor.

Possible side effects: When taken as directed, acetaminophen is usually not associated with side effects.

Be aware: If you consume 3 or more alcoholic drinks per day, consult your doctor before taking acetaminophen. Mixing this medication with alcohol can cause liver damage.

Tylenol Arthritis Pain

Generic name:
Acetaminophen

Other brand name(s):
Anacin (aspirin-free), Excedrin caplets, Panadol, Tylenol

Type of Medication: Analgesic (OTC)

What it's used for: To relieve pain in any form of arthritis

Dosage: 1,300 mg every 8 hours as needed; no more than 3,900 mg in 24 hours

Special instructions: Do not use with any other product containing acetaminophen; do not use for more than 10 days for pain – unless directed by a doctor.

Possible side effects: When taken as directed, acetaminophen is usually not associated with side effects.

Be aware: If you consume 3 or more alcoholic drinks per day, consult your doctor before taking acetaminophen. Mixing this medication with alcohol can cause liver damage.

Tylenol with Codeine #3

Generic name:
Acetaminophen with Codeine

Other brand name(s):
Phenaphen with Codeine

Type of medication: Analgesic

What it's used for: Pain not relieved by plain acetaminophen

Dosage: 15 to 60 mg every 4 hours as needed

Special instructions: Never take more of this drug than your doctor prescribes, because high doses of this drug can slow down breathing.

Possible side effects: Constipation, dizziness, lightheadedness, nausea, sedation, shortness of breath, vomiting

Be aware: If you consume 3 or more alcoholic drinks per day, consult your doctor before taking acetaminophen. Mixing this medication with alcohol can cause liver damage. Over time, this drug may cause psychological and physical dependence. Before taking this drug, let your doctor know if you use central nervous system depressants, such as antihistamines (allergy medications), tranquilizers, sleeping medications, muscle relaxants or narcotic pain medication, or if you have one of the following: liver disease, or history or alcohol or drug abuse.

Ultram

Generic name:
Tramadol

Type of medication: Analgesic

What it's used for: Severe pain from arthritis, fibromyalgia, surgery or fractures

Dosage: 50 to 100 mg every 4 to 6 hours as needed

Special instructions: Do not increase your dose on your own; do not stop abruptly unless advised to do so by your doctor; do not drive or operate heavy machinery until you know how your body reacts to this drug.

Possible side effects: Constipation, diarrhea, dizziness, drowsiness, increased sweating, loss of appetite, nausea

Be aware: Over time, this drug may cause psychological and physical dependence. Before taking this drug, let your doctor know if you use a central nervous system depressant, such as antihistamines (allergy medications), tranquilizers, sleeping medications, muscle relaxants or narcotic pain medications, or if you have one of the following: liver disease, or history of alcohol or drug abuse.

Ultracet

Generic name:
Tramadol with acetaminophen

Type of medication: Analgesic

What it's used for: Severe pain from arthritis, fibromyalgia, surgery or fractures

Dosage: 75 mg tramadol every 4 to 6 hours as needed for up to 5 days (no more than 600 mg per day)

Special instructions: Do not increase your dose on your own; do not stop abruptly unless advised to do so by your doctor. Do not take with other medications containing acetaminophen. Do not drive or operate heavy machinery until you know how your body reacts to this drug.

Possible side effects: Constipation, diarrhea, dizziness, drowsiness, increased sweating, loss of appetite, nausea

Be aware: If you consume 3 or more alcoholic drinks per day, consult your doctor before taking this medication. Mixing acetaminophen with alcohol can cause liver damage.

Over time, this drug may cause psychological and physical dependence. Before taking this drug, let your doctor know if you use a central nervous system depressant, such as antihistamines (allergy medications), tranquilizers, sleeping medications, muscle relaxants or narcotic pain medications, or if you have one of the following: liver disease, or history of alcohol or drug abuse.

Vicodin

Generic name:
Hydrocodone with acetaminophen

Other brand name(s):
Dolacet, Hydrocet, Lorcet, Lortab

Type of medication: Analgesic

What it's used for: Pain not relieved by plain acetaminophen

Dosage: 2.5 to 10 mg every 4 to 6 hours as needed

Special instructions: Do not increase dose on your own because side effects increase and tolerance develops as dosage increases; do not stop abruptly unless advised to do so by your doctor; do not drive or operate heavy machinery until you know how your body reacts to this drug.

Possible side effects: Constipation, dizziness, lightheadedness, mood changes, nausea, sedation, shortness of breath, vomiting and urinary retention

Be aware: If you consume 3 or more alcoholic drinks per day, consult your doctor before taking acetaminophen. Mixing this medication with alcohol can cause liver damage. Over time, this drug may cause psychological and physical dependence. Before taking this drug, let your doctor know if you use central nervous system depressants, such as antihistamines (allergy medications), tranquilizers, sleeping medications, muscle relaxants or narcotic pain medication, or if you have one of the following: liver disease, or history or alcohol or drug abuse.

Voltaren

Generic name:
Diclofenac sodium

Other brand name(s):
Voltaren-XR

Type of medication: NSAID

What it's used for: To control arthritis pain and inflammation

Dosage: 100 to 200 mg per day in 2 or 4 doses

Special instructions: Do not take with other prescription or OTC NSAIDs. Take as directed at the same times every day. If stomach upset occurs, take with food, a glass of milk or an antacid.

Possible side effects: Abdominal or stomach cramps, pain or discomfort; diarrhea; dizziness; edema (swelling of the feet); headache; gastrointestinal bleeding; heartburn or indigestion; nausea or vomiting; peptic ulcer

Be aware: Before taking this medication, let your doctor know if you drink alcohol or use blood thinners, or if you have or have had any of the following: sensitivity or allergy to aspirin or similar drugs, kidney or liver disease, heart disease, high blood pressure, asthma or stomach ulcers. Because stomach ulcers or internal bleeding can occur without warning, regular checkups are important. Patients on long-term NSAIDs should have blood counts and liver enzymes checked periodically. With diclofenac, liver enzymes should be checked within 4 to 8 weeks of starting the drug.

Unlike low-dose aspirin, there is little evidence that this or other NSAIDs will protect against heart attack or stroke. NSAIDs may be used with low-dose aspirin, but doing so may slightly increase your risk of gastric bleeding. Before taking this or any NSAID, tell your doctor if you take ACE inhibitors, lithium, warfarin or furosemide.

All NSAIDs may cause an increased risk of serious blood clots, heart attacks and stroke, which can be fatal. This risk may increase with dose and duration of use. Patients with cardiovascular disease or risk factors for cardiovascular disease may be at higher risk. These drugs should not be used for pain in people having coronary bypass surgery.

Voltaren-XR

Generic name:
Diclofenac sodium

Other brand name(s):
Voltaren

Type of medication: NSAID

What it's used for: To control arthritis pain and inflammation

Dosage: 100 mg per day in a single dose

Special instructions: Do not take with other prescription or OTC NSAIDs. Take as directed at the same time every day. If stomach upset occurs, take with food, a glass of milk or an antacid.

Possible side effects: Abdominal or stomach cramps, pain or discomfort; diarrhea; dizziness; edema (swelling of the feet); gastrointestinal bleeding; headache; heartburn or indigestion; nausea or vomiting; peptic ulcer

Be aware: Before taking this medication, let your doctor know if you drink alcohol or use blood thinners, or if you have or have had any of the following: sensitivity or allergy to aspirin or similar drugs, kidney or liver disease, heart disease, high blood pressure, asthma or stomach ulcers. Because stomach ulcers or internal bleeding can occur without warning, regular checkups are important. Patients on long-term NSAIDs should have blood counts and liver enzymes checked periodically.

Unlike low-dose aspirin, there is little evidence that this or other NSAIDs will protect against heart attack or stroke. NSAIDs may be used with low-dose aspirin, but doing so may slightly increase your risk of gastric bleeding. Before taking this or any NSAID, tell your doctor if you take ACE inhibitors, lithium, warfarin or furosemide. With diclofenac, liver enzymes should be checked within 4 to 8 weeks of starting the drug.

All NSAIDs may cause an increased risk of serious blood clots, heart attacks and stroke, which can be fatal. This risk may increase with dose and duration of use. Patients with cardiovascular disease or risk factors for cardiovascular disease may be at higher risk. These drugs should not be used for pain in people having coronary bypass surgery.

Zyloprim

Generic name:
Allopurinol

Other brand name(s):
Lopurin

Type of Medication: Uric-acid-lowering drug

What it's used for: Gout

Dosage: 100 to 800 mg per day in a single dose. The dose is adjusted to achieve a serum uric acid level lower than 6 mg/dl.

Special instructions: Take immediately after a meal. Stop taking at the first sign of a rash, which may indicate an allergic reaction.

Possible side effects: Skin rash, hives or itching

Be aware: Before taking this drug, let your doctor know if you use azathioprine (*Imuran*) or if you have kidney disease. Acute gout attacks are common when this drug is started. These attacks can be minimized by taking lower doses and by taking the drug with colchicine or NSAIDs. Never start or stop allopurinol during a flare.

Arthritis Resources

and Index

RESOURCES FOR GOOD LIVING

The Arthritis Foundation, the only national, voluntary health organization that works for the more than 46 million Americans with doctor-diagnosed arthritis, offers many valuable resources through more than 150 offices nationwide. Your local chapter has information, products, classes and other services to help you take control of your arthritis or related condition. To find the chapter office nearest you, call **(800) 568-4045** or search the Arthritis Foundation Web site at **www.arthritis.org**.

PROGRAMS AND SERVICES

- **Physician referral** – Most Arthritis Foundation chapters can provide a list of doctors in your area who specialize in the evaluation and treatment of arthritis and arthritis-related diseases.

- **Exercise programs** – The Arthritis Foundation sponsors, develops and coordinates exercise programs for people with arthritis, featuring specially-trained instructors. They include:

  1) Walk With Ease – This course allows participants to develop a walking plan that meets their individual needs, accompanied by the Arthritis Foundation book *Walk With Ease: Your Guide to Walking for Better Health, Improved Fitness and Less Pain.* An audio walking guide is now available to use during your walking routines, with guidelines, upbeat music and inspiring motivation. In addition, a

Walk With Ease group leader's manual is available to help you start and lead a walking group in your area.

2) Arthritis Foundation Exercise Program – Relieve stiffness and lessen arthritis pain by doing low-impact exercises designed for people with arthritis and taught by trained instructors.

3) Arthritis Foundation Aquatic Program – Join in the fun of a six- to 10-week exercise program in an heated pool led by trained instructors.

4) Arthritis Foundation Self-Help Program – Learn how to take control of your own care in this six week (15-hour) class for people with arthritis. This program was developed at Stanford University.

INFORMATION AND PRODUCTS

Find the latest information about arthritis, including research, medications, government advocacy, programs and services through one of the many information resources offered by the Arthritis Foundation:

- **www.arthritis.org** – Information about arthritis is available 24 hours a day on the Internet at the Arthritis Foundation's interactive, comprehensive Web site. Find news about arthritis, ways to get involved, and a variety of useful arthritis products, including books, brochures, videos and more.

- **Arthritis Answers** – Call toll-free at (800) 568-4045 for 24-hour, automated information about arthritis and Arthritis Foundation resources. Trained volunteers and staff are also available at your local Arthritis Foundation chapter to answer questions or refer you to physicians and other resources. Or email questions to help@arthritis.org.

- **Books** – The Arthritis Foundation publishes a variety of books on arthritis to help you learn to understand and manage your condition, live a healthier life, and cope with the emotional challenges that come with a chronic illness. Order books directly at www.arthritis.org or by calling (800) 283-7800. All Arthritis Foundation books are available at your local bookstore.

- **Brochures** – The Arthritis Foundation offers brochures containing concise, understandable information on the many arthritis-related diseases and conditions. Topics include surgery, the latest medications, guidance for working with your doctors and self-managing your illness. Single copies are available free of charge at www.arthritis.org or by calling (800) 568-4045.

- *Arthritis Today* – This award-winning bimonthly magazine provides the latest information on research, new treatments, trends and tips from experts and readers to help you manage arthritis. A one-year subscription to *Arthritis Today* is included when you become a member of the Arthritis Foundation. Annual membership is $20 and helps fund research to find cures for arthritis. Call (800) 283-7800 for information.

- ***Kids Get Arthritis Too*** – This newsletter focusing on juvenile rheumatic diseases, is published six times a year. Features speak to children and teens with the illness as well as to their parents. Stories examine the latest news in diagnosis, treatment and research of children's rheumatic diseases, as well as helpful ways kids can cope with their illnesses and the challenges they bring. This newsletter is free. To sign up, e-mail kgatmail@arthritis.org or write *Kids Get Arthritis Too*, 1330 West Peachtree Street, Suite 100, Atlanta, GA 30309.

Index

A

Abatacept, 68, 95, 256

Acetaminophen, 18, 39, 61-62, 96, 112, 187, 268, 317, 318
    with codeine, 97, 272, 319
    interactions with, 33

Active ingredients in label information, 20-21

Activella, 180

Actonel, 71, 98, 298
    with calcium, 99, 299

Actron, 57, 100-101, 214, 257, 259, 260

Adalimumab, 68, 101-2, 200

Adapin, 73
    interactions with, 31, 34

Advil, 18, 56, 103-4, 208, 242, 244, 253

Alendronate, 69, 71, 104-5, 196
    interactions with, 33
    with vitamin D, 105-6, 197

Aleve, 18, 57, 106-8, 115, 250

Allergies,
    telling doctor about, 23

Allopurinol, 74, 75, 108, 220, 328
    interactions with, 31, 33, 35

Alosetron hydrochloride, 79

Alternate-day therapy, 65

Ambien,
    interactions with, 34

American Association of Retired Persons (AARP), 51

American College of Rheumatology (ACR), 61, 62, 63

American Health-System Pharmacists, 85

American Society of Health-System Pharmacists, x, 84

Amigesic, 109, 112, 167, 227, 304

Amiloride,
    interactions with, 33

Amitriptyline, 72
    interactions with, 31

Amitriptyline hydrochloride, 73, 110, 178

Amitryptiline,
    interactions with, 34

Amphetamines,
    interactions with, 34

Anacin, 111, 122, 127, 131, 176, 188
    aspirin-free, 96, 112, 187, 268, 317, 318

Anaflex 750, 109, 112-13, 167, 227, 240, 304

Anakinra, 68, 113-14, 216

Analgesics, 61-62, 72, 96-97, 112, 124-25, 153-55, 170-71, 187, 201-2, 221-23, 241-42, 254-55, 263-68, 271-72, 286, 287, 302, 312-13, 317-21, 324

Anaprox, 106, 115-16, 250

Anaspaz, 80

Androgens, cyclosporine
    interactions with, 33

Angiotensin-converting enzyme (ACE) inhibitors, 104

Ankylosing spondylitis (AS), 66
    defined, 8
    medications for, 126, 182-83, 212-14, 294-95

Ansaid, 114-15, 194

Antacids,
    interactions with, 31, 35

Anthralin, 79

Anti-anxiety medications
    coffee and, 37-38
    grapefruit juice and, 37

Antibiotics, 41

Anticholinergic (antispasmotic) drugs, 79-80

Anticoagulant medications, 80

Antidepressants, 73, 110, 151-52, 171-72, 179, 288
    interactions with, 34

Antifungal medications,
    interactions with, 33

Antihistamines, 18, 97
    grapefruit juice and, 37

Antihypertensives,
    interaction with, 31

Anti-inflammatories, 144

Anti-malarial drugs,
    interactions with, 33

Antiphospholipid antibody syndrome, medications for, 80